The Alkal
Cookbook
3 in 1 BOX SET

Alkaline Breakfast, Lunch & Dinner Recipes for Health, Wellness& Weight Loss

By Marta Tuchowska

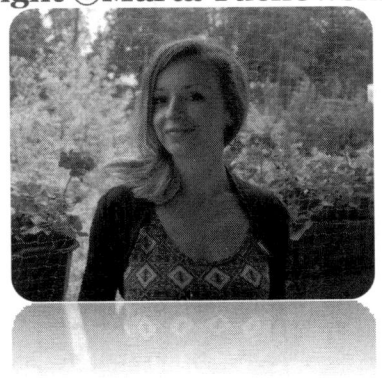

www.HolisticWellnessProject.com
www.amazon.com/author/mtuchowska

All cooking is an experiment in a sense, and many people come to the same or similar recipe over time. All recipes in this book have been derived from author's personal experience. Should any bear a close resemblance to those used elsewhere, that is purely coincidental.

IMPORTANT

The book is not intended to provide medical advice or to take the place of medical advice and treatment from your personal physician. Readers are advised to consult their own doctors or other qualified health professionals regarding the treatment of medical conditions. The author shall not be held liable or responsible for any misunderstanding or misuse of the information contained in this book. The information is not intended to diagnose, treat or cure any disease.

It is important to remember that the author of this book is not a doctor/ medical professional. Only opinions based upon her own personal experiences or research are cited. THE AUTHOR DOES NOT OFFER MEDICAL ADVICE or prescribe any treatments. For any health or medical issues – you should be talking to your doctor first.

The Alkaline Diet Lifestyle Cookbook

Introduction
The Amazing Benefits of the Alkaline Diet

Welcome to The Alkaline Diet Lifestyle Cookbook 3 in 1 BOX SET where it's all about healthy and nutritious alkaline recipes that are easy to prepare and will give you the energy you deserve. They will also help you understand the basics of the alkaline diet and lifestyle - even if you have never heard about Alkalinity before. It's focused on keeping things as simple and practical as possible.

This book is for you if:
-you feel like you want to have more energy for life
-you want to learn healthy cooking but don't know where to start
-you are vegan/vegetarian or you simply enjoy vegan inspired meals
-you are looking for a natural way to lose weight while giving your body the nutrition it needs
-you want to reduce the intake of animal products but don't know how to create recipes that you actually enjoy
-you want to transition towards a natural, wholesome, anti-inflammatory diet
-you don't want to spend hours in the kitchen yet want to be able to conjure up healthy and delicious meals that support your health and wellness goals

The Alkaline Diet- The Common Sense Approach

The alkaline diet is a lifestyle that encourages you to give your body the nourishment it needs so that it can work for you at its optimal levels without feeling too exhausted or too acidic. Too much acidity in the body is leading to depression, sickness, and obesity.

Dr. Robert O' Young, Director of Research at the pH Miracle Living Center, says that your fat may be protecting your very life against the acidity in your body. He goes on to make this bold statement.

"There is only one disease: The Constant Acidification of the Body."

What this means is that every disease, including excess weight, is because of a body that is too acidic. These things can make your body too acidic: processed foods, sugar, foods containing gluten and yeast, too much meat and animal products, stress, alcohol, tobacco, drugs, caffeine, and pollution.

Luckily, the alkaline diet gives us natural tools to fix the problem. I am not talking about overpriced superfoods from overseas that are difficult to find and to pronounce. The simplest methods are always the best and you will be surprised by how healthy you will feel by adding more everyday healing, alkaline foods into your diet (even if you don't follow a strict alkaline diet - there is no reason to go to the extreme - balance is the key to success).

If you attend the root cause of the problem, by implementing a lifestyle rich in alkaline forming foods, it will naturally take care of what plagues you.

My editor, Claire, is a 41-year-old professional woman and a single mom of 3 who suffered from obesity for many years.

She just did not have time to commit to a complicated weight loss program. She made many poor food choices because she was always pressed for time. As a result of her overly acidic body, she experienced tremendous pain from gastric reflux, so much so that her doctor wanted to operate on her.

But once she started following an alkaline diet (clean, moderate alkaline diet, nothing too strict), she stopped having gastric reflux pain. She began losing weight, and all without feeling deprived and without overdoing or overthinking it. She found she had more energy to get more done each day.

Here are a few simple guidelines that will help you transition towards a healthy, alkaline lifestyle. These are compatible with different nutritional lifestyles (Paleo, Gluten Free, Vegetarian, Vegan) and it's totally up to you what you choose to focus on:

1) **Eliminate processed foods from your diet and say "no" to colas and sodas** - there are so many additives and preservatives in these foods. They have been known to create hormone imbalances, make you tired, and add to acidity in your body. It's just not natural for humans to consume those conveniently processed foods. The label may even say "low in calories or low in fat"- it will not help you in your long term weight loss or health efforts. In order to start losing weight naturally, your body needs foods that are jam-packed with nutrients. Real foods. Living foods. This, in turn, will help your body maintain its optimal pH (7.35) almost effortlessly.

2) **Add more raw foods into your diet**- especially lots of vegetables and leafy greens as well as fruits that are naturally low in sugar (for example, limes, lemons, grapefruits, avocados, tomatoes, and pomegranates are alkaline forming fruits).

3) **Reduce animal products** – when and if you decide to consume them, make sure you choose organic meats and eggs, fresh fish, and always serve it with plenty of alkaline foods (for example salad or vegetables). Vegetables should comprise about 3 quarters of your plate.

4) **Drink plenty of clean, filtered water**, preferably alkaline water or fruit-infused water.

5) **Add more vegetable juices into your diet**- these are a great way to give your body more nutrients and alkalinity that will result in more energy, less inflammation and, if desired- natural weight loss. Vegetable juices are the best shots of health! I have written a bestselling book on <u>alkaline juicing</u> if want to give it a try and want to juice the right way.

6) **Reduce/eliminate processed grains, "crappy carbs" as well as yeast** (very acid-forming). Personally, I recommend quinoa instead (it's naturally gluten-free), amaranth (very nutritious), brown rice, or soba noodles (it's made from buckwheat and naturally gluten-free). You can also use gluten-free wraps or make your own bread (there are so many vegan and paleo bread recipes out there, you can pick and choose).

7) **Reduce/eliminate caffeine**- trust me - it will only make you feel sick and tired in the long run, and can even lead to adrenal exhaustion (not the best condition to end up in - I have been there). It may seem a bit drastic at first, and yes, I know what you're thinking- there are so many articles out there praising benefits of caffeine and coffee. Yes, I am sure there are, as many people build their business around coffee. This is why there must be something out there that promotes it. At the same time, I agree that everything is good for you in moderation. As long as you have a healthy foundation, you can have coffee as a treat (I do drink coffee

occasionally). There is no reason to be too strict on yourself. But...don't rely on caffeine as your main source of energy. Green tea may be helpful too as a transition, but green tea is not caffeine-free either so don't overdo it. On the other side of spectrum - green tea is rich in antioxidants and a great part of a balanced diet, so it's not that you have to get paranoid about all kinds of caffeine. <u>Moderation is the key</u>. Try to observe your body. Personally, I have noticed that quitting my coffee habits (I used to have 2-3 coffees a day) and replacing coffee with natural herbal teas and infusions have really made my energy levels skyrocket. Now I sleep better, and I get up feeling nice and fresh. I don't need caffeine to keep me awake. I no longer suffer from tension headaches and I feel calmer. Yes, I do have a cup of coffee as a treat sometimes, usually when I meet with a friend, but I no longer depend on it. I choose it; it doesn't choose me. Think about this and how you can apply this simple tip to your life to achieve total wellbeing. Coffee and caffeine in general is extremely acid-forming.

8) **Replace cow's milk with almond milk, coconut milk or any other vegan milk** (for example quinoa milk) that works well for you. Cow's milk is extremely acid forming and personally, I don't think it makes sense for humans to drink milk that is naturally designed for fattening baby calves not humans. Actually, quitting dairy was one of the best things I have done for myself. I have noticed that even very little milk would cause digestive problems and it was really easy to fix-I quit drinking milk. This is what all vegans and paleo diet followers say - dairy-free lifestyle is amazing!

9) **Don't fear good fats- coconut oil, olive oil, avocado oil** etc. are good for you and should replace processed margarines, and artery-clogging trans-fats.

   Also...

Use stevia instead of processed sugar (stevia is sweet but sugar-free) and Himalayan salt instead of regular salt (Himalayan salt contain some amounts of calcium, iron, potassium and magnesium plus it also contains lower amounts of sodium than regular salt.)

Add more spices and herbs into your diet- not only do they make your dishes taste amazing but they also have anti-inflammatory properties and help you detoxify (cilantro, turmeric, and cinnamon are miraculous).

As you can see, the alkaline diet is a pretty common sense clean diet. Nothing is exaggerated. Nothing is too strict. Nothing is too faddish. Eat more living foods and avoid processed foods. Try to eat more vegan/vegetarian (even if you are not 100% vegan).

Add regular relaxation techniques to the alkaline diet (including yoga, meditation), time spent in nature, adequate sleep and physical activity (we need to sweat out those toxins) and you have a prescription for health. It's strange to me that there are so many people putting the alkaline diet down, however, the general guidelines I have mentioned above are common sense for a healthy lifestyle and I am sure your doctor would agree with it (more natural foods, less process crap, more relaxation, less stress). This is the gist of the alkaline diet lifestyle. This is what will make you feel nice and rejuvenated and achieve your ideal weight. The problem is that some people are not willing to take those small common sense steps and are looking for a "secret formula" something that will magically help them with no effort at all. I am not judging- I have been guilty of it as well. We all have!

The truth is that whatever changes you want to make in your life (this rule applies not only to health) can be hard as leaving one's comfort zone is difficult, but with time and practise it becomes easy and automatic. Holistic success is about applying what we already know and using the information to better our lives. This is what I call "the secret formula." Information in action.

I always say that I am very open-minded when it comes to different diets. I never claim that what I do is the only path to wellness and health. I prefer to provide you with information and inspiration so that you can create your own way and choose what works for you. Everyone is different. What I teach is based on the alkaline way of living I learned from Doctor Young. However, my alkaline diet may be a bit different than yours and we can still be doing it the right way.
You need to learn to listen to your body and be good on yourself.

Now, with that being said, simply try to adhere to the following recommendations - they will help you understand the gist of the alkaline diet without overwhelming you with complicated pH discussions.

You can easily get started today- simply by making some minor adjustments to your existing diet. Baby steps. I always try to make things simple and easy to apply. Once you apply it - you will feel the amazing benefits of Alkalinity and from there you will want to carry on.

The alkaline diet is not a diet but a lifestyle really. It encourages you to add more alkalizing foods and drinks into your diet so that your body can heal itself naturally. How?

Alkaline Diet Crash Course- Understand the Basics

The pH of most of our important cellular and other fluids (like blood) is actually designed to be at pH of 7.35 (slightly alkaline).

The body has an intricate system in place to always maintain that healthy, slightly alkaline pH level – no matter what you eat. This is an argument that many alkaline diet skeptics use and I get it. It's 100% true.

This is not the goal of the alkaline diet. We just can't make our blood's pH more alkaline or "higher." Our body tries to work really hard for us to help us maintain our ideal pH (7.35). We can't have a pH of 8 or 10. If we did we would be dead.

The entire focus of the alkaline diet is to give your body the nourishment and healing tools it needs to MAINTAIN that optimal 7.35 pH almost effortlessly.

If we fail to do so, we torture our body with an incredible stress! Yes- when the body has to constantly work overtime to detoxify all the cells and maintain our pH it finally succumbs to disease.

Let me just name a few cases of what can happen if we constantly eat an acidic diet (also called SAD - Standard American Diet) that is not supporting our body at all. Our body ends up sick and tired of working overtime and may manifest one or more of the following conditions:

-constant inflammation

-immune and hormone imbalance

-lack of energy, mental fog

-yeast and candida overgrowth

-digestive damage

-weakened bones (our body is forced to pull minerals like magnesium and calcium from our bones in order to maintain alkaline balance it needs for constant healing processes).

In summary, eating more alkaline foods helps support our body so that it can work for us at optimal levels while eating more acidic food doesn't help at all. The alkaline diet is not about magically raising our pH but helping our body rebalance itself by supporting its natural healing functions.

However, it's not only about what we eat - it's also about how we live and what we think. It's not just a diet; it's a lifestyle. If you want vibrant health and alkaline wellness, try to be outdoors more, meditate, laugh, spend time with family and friends, do things you enjoy so that you can de-stress, practise mindfulness...It's not only about nutrition.

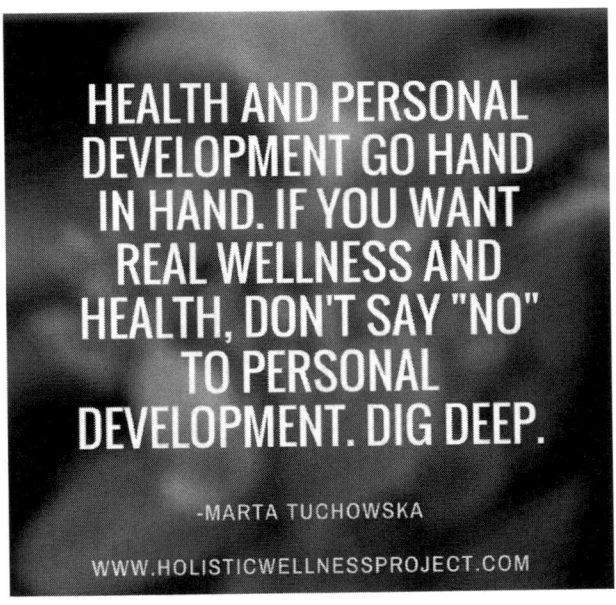

*Over the years, I have also learned that obsessing too much about food or health can be bad. I had to learn to let it go and focus on creating my healthy, alkaline lifestyle but at the same time **accepting occasional treats and cheats**. I had to learn to listen to my body and ignore some of the gurus' advice. You see - when you are too strict on yourself, this attitude takes away your emotional wellness. Balance is the key: we don't want to be too strict and too obsessed, but*

we don't want to end up being too lenient as well. You need to be honest with yourself and ask yourself what you can do better and reclaim responsibility for your health and wellness. It's always great to look for that next level, however it's also good to cultivate the sense of gratitude and accomplishment for what we have already managed to change in our diets and lifestyles.

Oftentimes, it's not about eating less - but about eating right.

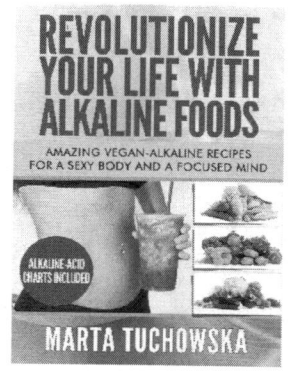

Never heard of the Alkaline Diet and don't know where to start?
I remember when I first learned about the alkaline diet. I was more than confused and sceptical. I wanted to take action but didn't know how. I would spend endless hours online looking for alkaline-acid charts only to find there was way too much contradictory information out there.

I don't want you to feel confused. I also really appreciate the fact you took an interest in my work. This is why I would love to offer you a free, complimentary 100 page e-book and **easy alkaline-acid charts** (printable so that you can keep them on your fridge or in your wallet). It will provide a solid foundation to kick-start your alkaline diet success. You will get all the facts explained in plain English, practical alkaline tips, and yummy, vegan-friendly recipes full of taste, motivational advice, as well as printable charts for quick reference. I will also show you how to combine the alkaline lifestyle with other diets (Paleo, vegetarian, vegan). The alkaline diet is very flexible, and it always welcome all kinds of "Alkalarians." You don't have to be 100% vegan to follow an alkaline diet, the choice is always yours.

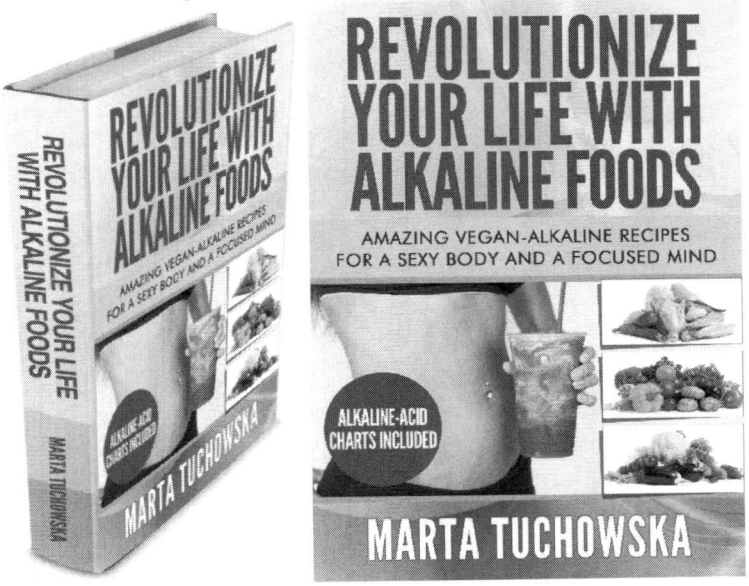

Visit the links below and grab your free copy of "How to Revolutionize Your Life with Alkaline Foods".
Download link:
www.holisticwellnessproject.com/alkaline-diet-ebook/giveaway.html

The benefits of eating more alkaline & plant-based foods

Since animal products are acid-forming, the alkaline diet is pretty vegan and plant-based in its design. But again- I am not telling you what to do. You will do what you want or feel you need to do. I always try to encourage people to try to stick with vegan options as much as possible- it's fun, it's creative and much more sustainable and better for our environment. However, you don't have to go 100% vegan unless you want to. Veganism and alkalinity very often overlap and many "alkalarians" are vegans or vegetarians, but we need to remember that vegans stick to their choices not only for their own health, but they also act against animal cruelty and climate changes. Some people go vegan for a variety of reasons including both their own health, environment, love for animals, energy, spiritual reasons etc.

To sum up - if you can't imagine yourself going vegan at this point, that's fine. Simply try to enrich your diet with more alkaline, plant-based options. This book will give you dozens of ideas to make a transition a really enjoyable experience. It's not very hard and you will feel healthier and energized as you eat more alkaline and less acidic. With the recipes you are just about to discover, I can guarantee that you won't feel deprived or bored. Having plenty of proven recipes is the key to success and the more you learn, the more motivated you will feel.

Also, remember that the recipes from this book can be changed and customized. Many of my readers, friends and clients are paleo diet enthusiasts yet they were able to skyrocket their energy levels, simply by following some of my alkaline tips and adding more alkaline foods and drinks into their diets.

Again we need to keep in mind that the alkaline diet is not about eating 100% alkaline. It's not about surviving on cucumbers and kale. Simply try to make about 70% of your diet rich in alkaline foods, while the remaining 30% can be acidic. Whenever in doubt, please check the charts that come as an additional, free resource with this book. You can download and print them at: www.bitly.com/AlkalineMarta

You may want to keep them at hand while shopping, or even going through my recipes.

About the recipes:

- Most ingredients are really easy, everyday and "common sense" ingredients that are easy to find at your local grocery store or supermarket. Occasionally, I may give you some recommendations for natural food supplements or some unusual super foods, but these are not the only path to wellness. The reason why I mention them is for informative purposes, in case you wish to add some new stuff into your diet or you simply like experimenting.
- You don't need to be a good cook or a qualified chef to learn those simple and delicious recipes. Honestly, I have never been "spend all her free time in her kitchen" girl (of course there is nothing wrong with that if you are absolutely passionate about cooking, but most people are too tired or too pressed for time). While I do enjoy cooking, as I am attracted to the *creative* part of it as well as health benefits that I can rip off if I cook the right way, I always try to make the whole process as simple as possible. I am a big fan of automation as well and so I like batch-cooking to make sure I always have some healthy options to fall, back on. Let's be real - everyone can have a bad day and cooking may seem like a mission. This is why having something that is already waiting for you that you prepared in advance is a great life saver. This is especially true if you are on a busy schedule or have a big family to feed.

- You don't need any fancy kitchen equipment to get started on my recipes. While having a good blender or food processor helps and so does food spiralizer (I recommend the brand Yanu Kitchen- YanuKitchen.com – you can grab it from Amazon), you can also use a simple hand blender and a knife. Add to it chopping boards, oven, pans and pots and you have all you need.
- Most of my recipes are quick to prepare- give it 20 minutes or less and you have a delicious and nutritious meal that supports your health and fitness goals.
- Since the alkaline diet is pretty vegan in its design, most of my recipes are also vegan. However, you can personalize them and you can easily include some meat or fish if you want to. Also, some of my recipes are Paleo friendly, (vegan-paleo to be **specific**- what a nice category) and they are very easy to be personalized. It's totally up to you if you want to transition your diet towards a vegan-vegetarian direction, which is my personal recommendation, but of course, it depends on your personal choices and to what extent you want to do it. This is why, aside from vegan recipes, you will also find a bonus section with simple, alkaline-paleo recipes that can help you make a transition. Again, let's remember that the alkaline diet is not about eating 100% alkaline. Let's aim for 70%. It's so much easier, right? The remaining 30% can be acidic foods, but this not justify processed foods that need to be buried forever. Your number one goal should be to eliminate all processed convenience foods. Then keep trying different foods and recipes and observe what works for you.

I always say that you need to listen to your body. On top of that, any drastic changes in your diet should be discussed with your doctor.

The Alkaline Diet Made Easy. Even for Busy People

As soon as you try my recipes and eat more alkaline, you will soon start noticing all the benefits of eating a diet jam-packed with vitamins, minerals, natural protein, fibre, healthy fats as well as free of sugar, gluten and artificial processed foods.

Now, here's why many people fail with the alkaline diet and healthy eating in general. I am not judging as I have been guilty of it many times. It stems from the fact that a person gets passionate about health, but tries to do it all at once or doesn't know where to start. You need a good strategy to fall back on.

It's simple, if you only rely on willpower your goals probably are:
-just ignore all the cravings and hold on
-eat only healthy alkaline foods and be strong and stick to it- if I have to survive on salads so be it!
-stop eating all the unhealthy stuff all at once

Unfortunately, this strategy is not a plan I recommend. It may not last for too long unless you are a super strong-willed person.

Here's the problem with this approach and I have faced it so many times:

You end up eating the same stuff all the time, and you get obsessed about foods. So you stress too much about the whole healthy eating thing. It means that you are constantly wondering what you're going to eat or what you just ate. Anxiety and guilt trips form part of this self-torture and it seems like health and wellness success is farther and farther away.

Then you think about your family and friends. They think you're a rabbit! They eat some yummy stuff and you are right in front of them with another boring salad (let me guess-iceberg lettuce, tomatoes and cucumber?).

It's not hard to fail in this scenario. In fact it's pretty normal. It would be weird if you didn't fail while following this crazy strategy. The risks could be that you don't get proper nutrition you need (you just worry too much about your pH) and your emotional wellness just leaves you.

The good news is that Marta is here to show you how to do it right with her recipes so that you eat a clean, balanced diet inspired by the alkaline diet and compatible with your current nutritional lifestyle. You enjoy it and so it's not that hard for you to create a healthy lifestyle. Moreover, it's cool to get new skills in the kitchen and treat your family and friends to healthy and delicious meals.

Alkaline Diet- Common Questions

Are lemons acidic or alkaline?
This is my favourite question and if you are a beginner, it's normal you are asking it. The answer is very simple: it's all about the effect that the food has on our body after it has been consumed, not before. It doesn't matter to us what pH they have in their natural state (before they have been eaten). Lemons are full of alkaline minerals and at the same time they don't contain sugar which makes them one of the very few alkaline fruits.
Remember to get your starter's guide and food list at:
www.bitly.com/AlkalineMarta
They will save you confusion.

What about Protein?
The choice to avoid/reduce the consumption of meat and other animal-derived products is becoming increasingly accepted among the general public. Restaurants and supermarkets are catering for vegans and those opting for an

alkaline diet or for those who want to eat more vegan or simply go dairy-free ever more than in the past offering a wide selection of delicious and vegan-friendly products. Some of these foods have been crafted to imitate certain things that you may wish to continue to enjoy, just in a novel, plant-based form, instead. Such things include non-dairy ice cream and yogurt, for example. Other foods, of course, are naturally vegan-friendly with even their conventional forms being entirely of plant origin.

Although the issue of finding vegan-friendly, alkaline products and restaurant items is becoming less of a problem in big cities and healthy food stores, this does not mean that this availability translates into a simple and easy life of making everyday vegan dishes at home. It's this particular challenge that we are now going to tackle with the help of the book you now hold in your hands. Making tasty and nutritious alkaline friendly dishes at home doesn't need to be difficult or expensive, and you'll soon be able to use the recipes in this book to prove it to yourself once and for all.

First of all, it's worth thinking about the nutritional side of things. It is simply a fact that animal products can provide us with certain vitamins, minerals and other micronutrients that can be harder to source from plants, although it is by no means impossible to do so. As such, anyone who makes the decision to simply consume less animal products or go vegetarian or vegan, must ensure that they find an adequate supply of such things using plants. The recipes chosen for inclusion within this book have been selected specifically for their richness in these particular vitamins and minerals.

Although fruits and vegetables are highly nutritious, they often do not contain suitably high levels of protein. Fortunately, other groups of plant-based foods do contain reasonable levels of protein. These foods include, but are not limited to:
- Hemp (You can use hemp powder in your smoothies.)

- Green leafy veggies (One cup of cooked spinach has about 7 grams of protein. Kale is pretty much the same.)
- Quinoa (It has about 9 grams of protein per cup.)
- Almond Butter (It is great with gluten-free breads and wraps. Two tablespoons of almond butter is about 8 grams of protein.)
- Other choices include: lentils (great in salads) and chickpeas

As you can see, despite first appearances, an alkaline diet even in its vegan form can still be rich in protein. One of the most important things to consider when making vegan alkaline dishes is the need to include more than one source of plant protein in each meal. This ought to be done in order to ensure that you are getting a wide enough range of proteins to promote your good health rather than sabotage it. Although this might sound complicated, it can be as simple as serving beans alongside rice as is popular in Caribbean cuisine, for example.

HEALTH BENEFITS OF VEGAN/ALKALINE DIETS OR SIMILAR:
- lower cholesterol levels
-lower blood pressure,
-lower rates of Type 2 diabetes,
-lower risk of death from heart disease,
-lower overall cancer rates
-less acidity in the body
-natural weight loss
-clean skin
-healthier immune system
-improved digestion

Do I have to give up my favourite foods forever?
Luckily, you don't. The mere thought of having to give everything up is just unbearable, right? Don't try to be perfect. Focus on progress. For example, in my opinion, people do

much better if they try to be 70-80% awesome and 20-30% relaxed than if they try to be 100% perfect- all the time. This rule also applies to other goals, not only health.

Besides, if you try to be perfect, you may experience many negative emotions that are not healthy. In fact, stressing too much about food can be much worse than having an occasional non-alkaline treat. So I guess, it's better to have a treat as a treat, relax and then move on to your regular lifestyle which is the alkaline diet lifestyle.

Remember the 80% rule! You don't have to give up your life. You can still go out with friends and socialize. You can still have that glass of wine or an occasional coffee. Going out for dinner with friends? My tip: order a big salad or veggie cream on side and then choose your favourite dish and enjoy it. Remember to drink plenty of clean water, you can even ask for lemon infused water. Alcohol is highly acid-forming, but you can enjoy a couple of drinks on social occasions every now and then. I am not talking about getting drunk of course, but there is nothing wrong with having an occasional drink with a friend and having a laugh. The problem is when you feel you need a drink because you can't deal with stress or you need it to boost your confidence (I have been there, I am not judging). In that case, I recommend you resort to meditation, hypnosis, NLP, yoga, natural remedies, guided meditation (you can download Five Senses Guided Meditation I created for you at: www.holisticwellnessproject.com/meditation-audiobook/giveaway.html).
You can also check out my blog that is full of holistic wellness and relaxation tips:
www.HolisticWellnessProject.com

There are many options out there that can help you create a new, stronger, more stress-free and more confident version of yourself with long-term success.

So back to acidic foods and drinks, just remember-moderation is the key. It's not that you will have to give up all the acidic foods forever. At the same time, I am not saying you should be indulging in unhealthy foods all the time. Just follow your own pace.

However, I strongly recommend you give up sodas and other artificial drinks as well as chemically processed foods, burgers, fried and convenience foods. They do not bring you closer to your goals at all. There are healthier snacks out there, you can make your own fries and crisps, and you can experiment with fruit infused water that is a great alternative to sodas and also much, much cheaper.

Also don't try to do it all at once. Set simple goals. For example: this week I will replace sodas with fruit infused water. Action plan: get the recipes and ingredients. Done? Great. Next step. Repeat the process, for example: this week I will try to drink one alkaline smoothie a day and have some salad with my lunch/dinner. Done? Great. Create the next step. For example: this week, I will get committed to physical activity or yoga. Only one step at the time. Baby steps. Here and now. I call it- mindful motivation.

Are all the recipes from the Alkaline Diet Lifestyle Cookbook 100% vegan?

Yes, almost all of my recipes are vegan and some of them are paleo-vegan, meaning that they do not include any grains or legumes and can be easily customized (you can add other foods, but remember to keep about 70% of your plate full of alkalizing foods).

To sum up- the main part of this book are alkaline-vegan recipes. I also included a bonus at the end of this book. The bonus includes some alkaline-paleo friendly and alkaline-vegetarian recipes (not vegan), that I believe can be great for those who want to transition or simply enjoy all kinds of recipes. It's all about the 80/20% rule. Even 70/30% is fine to begin with. Aim to eat 70% alkaline.

Now, with all of that information out of the way, it's time to start looking at some delicious recipes. Each category includes a number of tasty dishes with a little description telling you what's so good about it from a nutritional/lifestyle point of view. You'll also find easy to follow instructions for each dish, so you'll never have a moment's hesitation when making beautiful and healthy dishes for you and your loved ones.

Shall you happen to have any questions or doubts about this book (or you want to say hi) just email me at: info@holisticwellnessproject.com
I love hearing from my readers!

Important:
I am not a doctor/therapist or a scientist, and I am not giving you any specific advice related to serious health problems. So if you happen to have any specific health questions, remember to talk to your doctor or health professional first. Please read a full disclaimer at the beginning of this book.

As a wellness coach I help people with **motivation**, habits and **practical holistic self-care tips** so that they can create a healthy lifestyle with long-term benefits that allows them to prevent numerous illnesses and lose weight in a healthy way. I call it a holistic lifestyle design, something that I am absolutely passionate about and honestly, I am even more passionate about helping you being passionate about it as well. This is my mission and this is what I stand for. I want to help you work on your body, mind and soul so that you can create success in all areas of life. It all starts with energy and vibrant health. You can also use my recipes as templates to create your own. If there is any ingredient you don't like or your body can't tolerate - skip it. We need to listen to our body and be selective if necessary. Everyone is different and so are their nutritional preferences. Follow your way.

Read on and enjoy!

Don't forget to download your free complimentary eBook at:

www.holisticwellnessproject.com/alkaline-diet-ebook/giveaway.html

You will automatically join my free alkaline newsletter meaning that you will be notified about my new books during the pre-launch stage (=you will be receiving them for free or only 99c.). Not to mention the insider news, tips, recipes and more healthy updates you will love.

Recipe Measurements

I love keeping ingredient measurements as simple as possible-this is why I stick to tablespoons, teaspoons and cups.

The cup measurement I use is the American cup measurement. I also use it for dry ingredients. If you are new to it, let me help you:

If you don't have American Cup measures, just use a metric or imperial liquid measuring jug and fill your jug with your ingredient to the corresponding level. Here's how to go about it:

1 American Cup= 250ml= 8 fl.oz

For example:

If a recipe calls for 1 cup of almonds, simply place your almonds into your measuring jug until it reaches the 250 ml/8oz mark.

I know that different countries use different measurements and I wanted to make things simple for you.

Translations (US-UK English)

Eggplant=Aubergine
Zucchini=Courgette
Cilantro=Coriander
Garbanzo Beans=Chickpeas
Navy Beans-=Haricot Beans
Aragula=Rocket
Broth=Stock

BOOK 1
The Alkaline Diet Lifestyle Cookbook Vol.1

Sensational Alkaline Breakfast Recipes for Natural Energy, Health, and Weight Loss

<u>Beautiful Alkaline-Diet-Inspired Clean Eating Breakfasts</u>

Breakfast can be one of the biggest challenges for new "alkalarians" as well as many people who want to get healthy. It may also be hard to adapt breakfasts if you have no idea how to make them both nice and quick as well as delicious and nutritious. However, it doesn't have to be this way. You are just about to discover that you have another option. Say goodbye to heavy breakfasts that are way difficult to digest and forget about skipping breakfasts with a cup of coffee (coffee is acid-forming, while it's OK as a little treat every now and then, it should not be abused).

<u>It's not about eating less or going hungry, it's about eating right</u>. You can enjoy a wide variety of clean meals composed of plenty of healing alkaline foods which will give you that morning boost you so desperately need. The recipes below are meant to give you an idea of the delicious, and yet simple, creations you can make every morning to fill your body with goodness so that it is ready for the day ahead.

Give yourself the energy you deserve first thing in the morning. If you start your day healthy, you will end your day feeling healthy! Whether you wake up craving sweetness or are planning to do some healthy baking to create some nice and guilt-free breakfast treats these recipes will give you both. If you need to have a solid breakfast because you wake up hungry, or are looking for a quick breakfast snack, raw food options or a takeaway breakfast you are about to discover a myriad of alkaline-friendly, clean diet recipes to pick and choose from depending on your mood and taste preferences. Choosing what you want to eat will make you feel better about eating a healthy, nutritious breakfast in the morning.

This is not a book on strict dieting, but a book on creating a healthy and balanced lifestyle through alkaline food inspired nutrition. My goal is to help you achieve long term success and help you spare frustration, fad diets and stress that you may experience when counting calories.

SECTION I
Porridges, Puddings, Pancakes, Bakes

Almost Alkaline Choco Porridge

Although chocolate doesn't sound like much of a breakfast, pure cocoa contains an extraordinarily high level of antioxidants and beneficial plant fats. We won't be using the typical chocolate you're thinking of; the one devoid of all nutrition. You can use cocoa powder to get all the beneficial effects of the delicious cocoa bean. Combined with almonds and quinoa, this recipe makes for a perfectly energy-dense morning boost. It is great for mental focus and concentration. Raw cocoa is not super alkaline, however this recipes balances it with more alkaline ingredients to create a super powerful breakfast for busy people. Yum!

Serves: 2
Ingredients:
- Half cup cooked quinoa
- 2 tbsp. raw cocoa powder, unsweetened
- 2 cups almond or coconut milk
- Handful of almonds, chopped
- Handful of dried cranberries or other fruit of your choice
- 2 tbsp. desiccated coconut
- 2 tbsp. raw almond butter, unsweetened
- 1 tbsp. ginger powder

Optional:
- 2 tbsp. barley grass powder for more alkaline benefits and nutrition
- 2 tbsp. chia seeds for more nutrition

Instructions:

1. Mix the quinoa and unsweetened cocoa powder in a breakfast cereal bowl(s).
2. Pour the coconut milk (or other plant-derived milk) into the bowl and mix well. If the mixture is too dry, add a little more.
3. It's best to cover this mixture and allow it to sit overnight. You don't have to do this if you would prefer not to, though.
4. Stir the mixture and then add the ginger powder, almonds and cranberries and other fruit of your choice.
5. Scatter the desiccated coconut over the top of the mixture and place the almond butter in the middle.
6. Give it all a quick stir and enjoy.

Alka Paleo Flax Seed Mix

Great option for breakfast on the go. It's all too common to run out the door without eating anything, but as soon as we do it, we end up grabbing whatever is available, and *not* making the best choices. Here is one of my favorites; simply blend all together and enjoy!

Serves: 2
Ingredients:
- 2 avocados, peeled, pitted and chopped
- 1 cup almond milk or coconut milk
- 1 tablespoon ground flax seeds (chia could work great here, too)
- ½ cup soy sprouts (I am not talking about soy, but soy sprouts)
- Olive oil and Himalayan salt to taste

Instructions:
Blend and enjoy!

Alkaline Panna Cotta

Panna Cotta is a traditional Italian dessert recipe that also makes a great breakfast meal. I was able to transform this recipe and make it dairy-free and vegan/alkaline friendly. If you want to enjoy it for breakfast, you will need to get into a habit of preparing it after dinner and let it form properly overnight. It will only take a few minutes to prepare and trust me - it will be easier for you to wake up and get up knowing that there is an amazing panna cotta waiting for you.

Serves: 2-3
Ingredients:
- 1 cup coconut milk
- 1 cup almond milk (unsweetened) - if you are allergic to almond, use coconut milk or organic rice milk instead (total 2 cups, if you want to use more milk, use more gelatin as well)
- 2 tablespoons of unflavored vegan-friendly Gelatin (Unflavored Vegan Gel)
- 2 tablespoons Stevia
- 2 teaspoons vanilla extract
- 2 teaspoons cinnamon powder
- Juice of 1 lemon
- 2 tablespoons chia seeds
- OPTIONAL: 2 TABLESPOONS BARLEY GRASS (it's jam-packed with nutrients)
- Toppings of your choice (maybe homemade marmalade or some fruit?)

Instructions:
1. Pour the milk mix into a saucepan and add in gelatin.
2. Whisk steadily for 5 minutes (no heat).
3. Then, add in stevia, cinnamon, vanilla, chia seeds and green powders (this is optional).
4. Turn on the heat (medium heat) and keep stirring constantly, until milk is hot enough to steam.
5. Important- Do not boil as this will deactivate the gelling properties of the gelatin.

6. Turn off the heat and leave to cool down for a few minutes.
7. In the meantime, grease small bowls with coconut oil and pour the heated mixture into the bowls.
8. Cover and place in the fridge for about 8 hours (yep...you have to wait 8 hours...that's the only drawback of this recipe)
9. When ready, serve directly in bowls (like I did here, nothing too artistic really - I was pressed for time) or gently turn them upside down on to a place and add toppings (this is what I am going to do for my special guests!)

Awesome Energy Bars

Great recipe for batch-cooking to make sure you always have a ready to grab healthy breakfast option!

Makes 5-6 bars
Ingredients:
- 1 banana, mashed
- 1/4 cup almonds
- 1/3 cup dried plums
- 1/4 cup sunflower seeds
- 1/4 cup vanilla or hemp protein powder
- 2 tbsp. arrowroot starch
- 1/2 cup almond flour

Instructions:
1. Combine mashed banana with almond flour and arrowroot starch.
2. Mix well and then add in dried plums, nuts, seeds, almond flour and protein powder. Place through a food processor.
3. Add mix to a pan greased with coconut oil and bake at 275 °F (130 °C) for about 30 minutes.
4. Remove and let cool then cut into bars or squares.
5. Enjoy!

Cinnamon Quinoa Bowl

Servings: 2
Ingredients:
- 1 cup uncooked quinoa
- 1 ½ cups water
- ½ teaspoon ground cinnamon
- Pinch of Himalayan salt

Instructions:

1. Rinse the quinoa well.
2. In a medium-sized saucepan, combine the quinoa, water, cinnamon and salt.
3. Bring to a boil.
4. Then, turn down the heat, cover, and simmer for 10 minutes.
5. When cooked, remove from the heat.
6. Cool down.
7. Serve drizzled with coconut or almond milk.
8. Enjoy!

Vegan Apple Cinnamon Muffins

Here comes another treat recipe. While alkaline diet tries to avoid sugar in all its forms, it's totally okay to use some stevia for natural sweetness (stevia is not sugar).

Servings: 12

Ingredients:
- 1 ½ tablespoon flaxseed meal
- 2 ½ tablespoons warm water
- 3 teaspoons coconut oil
- 2 large ripe apples, diced
- 1 cup unsweetened coconut milk
- ¾ cup lemon juice
- A few drops of stevia
- 3 tablespoons vegetable oil
- ½ tablespoon vanilla extract
- 1 ½ cups gluten-free flour blend
- 1 ½ teaspoon ground cinnamon
- 1 teaspoon baking soda
- Pinch of Himalayan salt
- ½ cup old-fashioned oats (gluten-free)

Instructions:
1. Preheat your oven to a temperature of 375°F (190 Celsius).
2. Line a muffin pan with paper liners.
3. Using a bowl, whisk the flaxseed and water together. Let rest for 10 minutes.
4. Heat the coconut oil over the medium heat (use a small saucepan)
5. Add the apples and toss them with cinnamon then cook for a few minutes until soft.
6. Remove the apples from heat.
7. Combine the almond milk, lemon juice, stevia, oil, and the vanilla extract in a mixing bowl.
8. Whisk in the flax mixture until it is super smooth.

9. In a separate bowl, mix together the gluten-free flour blend, cinnamon, and baking soda as well as Himalayan salt.
10. Mix the dry ingredients with the wet ingredients until smooth.
11. Carefully fold in the oats and the sautéed apples.
12. Place the batter into the prepared muffin pan, filling the cups completely.
13. Bake for about 20 minutes until a knife inserted in the center comes out clean.
14. Cool the muffins for 15-20 minutes, serve and enjoy!

Avocado Choco Mousse

If you like healthy treats for breakfast, be sure to prepare this one before you go to bed. Just like with the panna cotta, it needs some time to sit well.

Servings: 6 to 8
Ingredients:
- 1/2 cup cocoa powder
- 4 large ripe avocados, pitted and chopped
- ½ cup unsweetened almond milk
- 1 tablespoon pure vanilla extract
- A few drops of liquid stevia
- ¼ cup soaked almonds

Instructions:

1. In a blender or food processor, blend the mixture until smooth and well combined.
2. Spoon into dessert cups and chill for 4 to 6 hours before serving.
3. Enjoy!

Vegan Paleo-Friendly Porridge

This recipe is both alkaline and paleo friendly. It offers a highly energizing mix of seeds that is nicely alkalized by spices and lemon juice. It's a perfect breakfast for busy people. No excuses - don't skip breakfast.

Servings: 1

Ingredients:

- ¼ cup chopped walnuts
- 2 tablespoons pumpkin seeds
- 1 tablespoon raw chia seeds
- 1 teaspoon ground cinnamon
- 1 teaspoon nutmeg
- 1 cup almond milk or coconut milk
- 1 tablespoon of melted coconut oil
- Juice of 1 lemon
- Juice of 1 grapefruit
- Optional: 1 teaspoon of barley grass powder

Instructions:

1. Combine your ingredients in a cereal bowl and pour over some coconut or almond milk.
2. Stir well and serve.
3. Enjoy!

Amaranth Coconut Porridge

Amaranth is a great source of iron and of the healthiest of the grains there are. Personally, I prefer quinoa, but I like to switch to amaranth every now and then. Variety is the key. Both quinoa and amaranth are gluten-free and a spectacular addition to a balanced diet.

Servings: 2
Ingredients:
- 2 cups water
- 1 cup amaranth
- 1 cup coconut milk
- ½ cup shredded coconut, slightly toasted

Instructions:

1. Add amaranth to boiling water.
2. Reduce heat and simmer on medium heat for 15- 20 minutes until amaranth is cooked.
3. Remove from heat and stir in the coconut milk as well as the toasted coconut.
4. Add some stevia to sweeten if you wish (you can also serve it with some homemade marmalade) and enjoy!

Cinnamon Pumpkin Porridge

With a variety of porridge recipes in this book, there is no chance you will ever get bored. Here comes another delicious recipe with anti-inflammatory, alkalizing properties.

Servings: 2

Ingredients:

- 1 cup unsweetened almond milk or coconut milk
- 1 cup water
- 1 cup uncooked quinoa
- ½ cup pumpkin puree
- 1 teaspoon ground cinnamon
- 2 tablespoons ground flaxseed meal
- Juice of 1 lemon

Instructions:

1. Whisk together the water and almond milk.
2. Bring the mixture to boil.
3. Stir in the quinoa, pumpkin, and cinnamon.
4. Reduce the heat.
5. Cover and simmer for 10 minutes or until the liquid has been absorbed.
6. Remove from the heat and then stir in the flaxseed meal.
7. Place the porridge into small bowls.
8. Sprinkle some lemon juice and add some pumpkin seeds on top if desired.

Hemp Protein Crepes

Meat is not the only way to get protein, there are many other plant-based options out there and this recipe is the best proof of how you can combine taste and health.

Hemp seed is full of essential fats, antioxidants, amino acids, fiber, iron, zinc, carotene, vitamin B1, vitamin B2, vitamin B6, vitamin D, vitamin E, chlorophyll, calcium, magnesium, copper, potassium, phosphorus, and enzymes just to name a few. If you want to eat more vegan, make sure to add some hemp seeds into your diet.

Servings: 4 to 6

Ingredients:

- 3 cups of almond milk
- 2 tablespoons of coconut oil, melted
- 2 cups rice flour or almond flour
- ¼ cup hemp seeds (raw)
- 1 ripe banana, peeled and mashed
- Olive oil or coconut oil, as needed

Instructions:

1. In a mixing bowl, combine the almond milk, coconut oil, flour, and hemp seeds.
2. Whisk until well combined.
3. Add in the mashed banana – stir until lump-free.
4. Heat some olive oil or coconut oil using a small skillet (medium heat).
5. Pour in about ¼ cup of the batter and tilt the pan to coat the bottom well.
6. Cook for a few minutes or until the edges of the crepe are dry and nicely browned.
7. Flip carefully and cook on the other side.
8. Repeat the process to create more protein pancakes.
9. Enjoy!

Coconut Apple Choco Stir Fry

Craving something sweet? Here comes a perfect guilt-free solution that is also full of nutrition. As you may have noticed, I like barley grass powder a lot. It's full of nutrients and alkalizing properties.

Serves: 2
Ingredients:
- 2 green apples, peeled and chopped
- 1 tablespoons coconut oil
- 1 teaspoon cinnamon powder
- 2 tablespoons chia seeds
- Stevia to sweeten
- 2 tablespoons raw cocoa powder
- 1 tablespoon of barley grass

Instructions:
1. Heat up some coconut oil in a frying pan.
2. Add the apples, cinnamon, stevia and cook until soft.
3. Turn off the heat and add some raw cocoa and chia seeds.
4. Stir well.
5. Place in dessert bowls, sprinkle over some barley grass.
6. Cool down in a fridge, serve and enjoy!

Easy Anti Inflammatory Apple Treat

Sugar and artificial ingredients aggravate inflammation while living foods and spices help alleviate it. If you are looking for yummy breakfast ideas with anti-inflammatory properties this is the recipe for you.

Servings: 4 to 6
Ingredients:
- 1 ½ cups chopped apple
- ¼ cup lemon juice
- 1 ½ tablespoons coconut oil
- 1 ½ teaspoons ground cinnamon
- Stevia to sweeten

Instructions:

1. Combine the apples, cinnamon, coconut oil and lemon juice in a small saucepan.
2. Heat over medium heat and cook for a few minutes until tender.
3. Add some stevia to sweeten if you wish.
4. Serve with puddings, porridges, crepes or just as a natural treat with some seeds for more nutrition.
5. Enjoy!

Yummy Hazelnut Treat

Servings: 4 to 6

Ingredients:

- 2 cups of raw hazelnuts
- 2 tablespoons of unsweetened raw cocoa powder
- 1 teaspoon of pure vanilla extract
- 10 drops liquid stevia

Instructions:

1. Preheat your oven to a temperature of 375°F (190 °C).
2. Spread the hazelnuts on the baking sheet and roast for about 15 minutes.
3. Place the roasted nuts into a small metal mixing bowl.
4. If you wish, cool down and remove the skins.
5. Place the hazelnuts (minus the skins) in your food processor to blend into a powder.
6. Add the cocoa powder, vanilla extract, and stevia.
7. Place in a glass container and store in a fridge.
8. Serve with puddings, porridges, or as a snack. You can also serve it with some fruit.
9. Enjoy!

Tropical Granola

Another easy way to get your morning boost is to make a huge batch of delicious granola in advance. You can easily make some to enjoy every morning all week long. You'll get a healthy source of carbohydrates from the grains used, and you'll get plenty of fats and proteins from the combination of nutritious nuts and seeds.

Serves: 4

Ingredients:

- 1 tsp coconut oil
- 2 tbsp. stevia powder
- 1 tsp ginger powder
- 1 tsp vanilla extract
- 1 cup rolled oats (cooked quinoa or amaranth also works fine)
- 1/2 tsp cinnamon
- ¼ cup almonds, soaked
- ¼ cup pumpkin seeds
- ¼ cup desiccated coconut
- ¼ cup dried dates
- Coconut yogurt to mix in
- Juice of 1 lime (optional)

Instructions:

1. Preheat the oven to 300°F.
2. Whisk the coconut oil, stevia and vanilla extract to make a syrupy mixture.
3. Mix the rolled oats with the cinnamon and pour evenly onto a baking tray. Toast the rolled oats for 10 minutes in the oven.
4. Add the almonds, pumpkin seeds and some of the desiccated coconut and mix into the semi-toasted oats.
5. Add the syrup mixture to the oats, ensuring that everything is coated well.
6. Toast the mixture for a further 20 minutes or so.
7. Add the rest of the desiccated coconut and the dried dates. Mix well and allow to cool.
8. Store in a suitable airtight container. Serve alongside some vegan-friendly yogurt such as coconut yogurt.

Alka-Berry Pancakes

This is a perfect way to incorporate the healthfulness of berries with a classic breakfast like pancakes. I like to make some on a Sunday evening so that I have something to look forward on Monday morning when I have to be up early. Besides, it's nice to get up and have a ready to grab breakfast (also great as a take-away breakfast).

Makes approximately 8 pancakes

Ingredients:

- 1 1/4 cups almond flour
- 1 tsp. stevia
- 1 1/2 tsp. baking powder
- 1 tsp. bicarbonate of soda
- Dash of Himalayan salt
- 1/2 tsp. ground nutmeg
- 1 cup coconut milk
- 1 banana, mashed
- 1 tbsp. vegan butter or coconut oil
- 1 tbsp. olive oil
- Blueberries or pomegranates or grapefruits

Instructions:

1. Combine the flour, stevia baking powder, bicarbonate of soda, nutmeg and a dash of salt in a bowl.
2. Whisk the mashed banana into the coconut milk.
3. Make a well in the middle of the flour mixture and slowly add the milk mixture, folding it in gently as you go along. Leave the mixture to sit a while.
4. Melt the vegan butter or coconut oil and the olive oil in a nonstick pan over a medium heat.
5. Ladle a small amount of the pancake batter into the pan and allow each pancake to cook one at a time. Stack them one on top of the other when cooked, making sure that you put a little vegan butter between each layer to prevent them from sticking together.
6. Serve with blueberries, or some alkaline fruits like pomegranates or grapefruits. Enjoy!

Buckwheat and Banana Porridge

This recipe is great for cold winter mornings. It will keep you full till lunch!

Servings: 2
Ingredients:

- 1 cup water
- 1 cup buckwheat grouts
- 2 big grapefruits, peeled and sliced
- Stevia to sweeten (optional)
- 1 tablespoon ground cinnamon
- 3 to 4 cups of almond milk
- 2 tablespoons natural almond butter
- Optional: 1 tablespoon of barley grass green powder

Instructions:

1. Whisk together the water and buckwheat in a medium saucepan.
2. Bring the water to boil then add buckwheat.
3. Keep cooking till the buckwheat absorbs all the water.
4. Reduce heat and add in some almond milk. Stir well.
5. Add in the rest of the ingredients except grapefruit.
6. Turn of the heat and place into cereal bowls adding some grapefruit chunks.
7. Enjoy!

Almond Paleo Style Alka-Porridge

This is a perfect and Paleo friendly alternative for those who can't tolerate grains (even healthy grains). All you need to do is to...go nuts!

Servings: 2
Ingredients:

- 1 cup chopped almonds
- 1/3 cup shredded coconut, unsweetened
- 2 tablespoons pumpkin seeds (or any other seeds of your choice)
- 2 tablespoon chia seeds
- 1 tablespoon ground flaxseed
- 1 teaspoon ground cinnamon
- 1 teaspoon almond extract
- 2 cup boiling hot water
- Coconut yoghurt or cream to serve
- Homemade sugar-free marmalade to serve (check out the next recipe)

Instructions:

1. Place all the dry ingredients (except spices) though a blender until powdered.
2. Add in some hot water and stir well.
3. Finish off by adding spices, vegan yoghurt of your choice and home-made marmalade.
4. Enjoy!

Home-Made Anti-Inflammatory Marmalade

This recipe is not only a healthy alternative to processed marmalades that are full of sugar but it's also great to help you save some money whole creating a healthy and guilt-free with anti-inflammatory properties!

Serves: 2 cups of marmalade
Ingredients:
- 1 cup pineapple chunks (small)
- 1 cup grapefruit chunks (small)
- 1 tablespoon cinnamon
- 1 tablespoon fresh grated ginger (or ginger powder)
- ½ tablespoon nutmeg
- Optional: stevia to sweeten (just a few drips will do)
- 3-4 tablespoons of coconut oil
- ¼ cup coconut milk or cream (raw, unsweetened)

Instructions:
1. Heat up coconut oil in a pan over medium heat.
2. Add the fruits and keep stirring.
3. When the fruits get slightly soft, add the spices stirring well.
4. Keep adding some coconut milk or cream to add some nice flavours and softness.
5. Keep stirring for a few minutes or until the fruits are soft.
6. Cool down and place in jars.
7. Store in a fridge for a few hours or overnight before serving.
8. Great to serve with pancakes, puddings and other treats. I also like it on raw fruits like apples.
9. Enjoy! It's really healthy!

Green Cinnamon Apple Oats

Servings: 4

Oats Ingredients:

- 2 cups of unsweetened almond milk
- 2 cups boiling water
- 2 teaspoons of vanilla extract
- 2 cups of old-fashioned oats (gluten-free)
- 2 tablespoons of chia seeds
- 1 teaspoon of ground cinnamon
- 1 tablespoon alfalfa powder or barley grass green powder
- Juice of 1 lemon
- Optional: stevia to sweeten

Apple Topping:

- 2 tablespoons of coconut oil
- 2 medium apples, cored and chopped
- Stevia (optional)
- 1 teaspoon cinnamon powder

Instructions:

1. Place oats in a cereal bowl and add in the warm water. Stir well and cover.
2. In the meantime, heat up some coconut oil in a frying pan (medium heat). Add the apples and sauté until slightly soft.
3. When done, turn off the heat and combine the apples with the oats in the cereal bowl.
4. Add almond milk, chia seeds, vanilla and alfalfa powder.
5. Sweeten with stevia if you wish.
6. Sprinkle over some lemon juice.
7. You can also serve it with some homemade marmalade from the previous recipe.
8. Enjoy!

Variations- oats can be replaced by quinoa as well as crushed nuts and seeds (for example walnuts, cashews or almonds). Experiment to your heart's content.

Spicy Pumpkin 100% Vegan Muffins

I won't lie to you; this is not the best recipe if you are pressed for time. However, it may be worth trying on a Sunday evening to make sure you have a nice take-away breakfast for the next day.

Servings: 12
Ingredients:

- 1 tablespoons of ground flaxseed
- 1/2 cup of warm water
- 2/3 cups of rice flour
- ½ cup of buckwheat flour
- ½ cup of tapioca starch
- 1 teaspoon of pumpkin pie spice
- 1 teaspoon of baking soda
- ½ teaspoon of baking powder
- ½ teaspoon of Himalayan salt
- 1 ¼ cups of pumpkin puree
- Stevia to sweeten (optional)
- ½ cup of melted coconut oil
- ¼ cup of water, cold
- 1/3 cup finely chopped almonds

To serve:

-pomegranate fruits or grapefruit slices

Instructions:

1. First, preheat your oven to a temperature of 325°F (160 Celsius)
2. In the meantime, use paper liners to line the cups of a muffin pan.
3. Combine flaxseed and the water, whisk energetically and let the mixture rest for 10 minutes.
4. In a mixing bowl, combine rice flour with buckwheat flour.
5. Add the tapioca starch, pumpkin pie spice, baking soda, baking powder and Himalayan salt.

6. Take another bowl to mix the pumpkin puree with stevia, coconut oil, water, and the flaxseed mixture.
7. Stir the dry ingredient mixture into the wet ingredient mixture. Be sure there are no lumps.
8. Fold in the almonds. Spoon the muffin batter into the muffin pan, filling each cup.
9. Bake for about 40-45 minutes. Cool down and serve with some fruit, like for example alkaline fruit (grapefruit, pomegranate etc.)

Section II

Amazingly Delicious and Nutritious Smoothies and Juices

Nice and Fresh Mint Smoothie

This smoothie is great for digestion and is full of antioxidant properties. In addition, it helps you keep hydrated and nicely refreshed. Personally, I find the mint really effective in alleviating headaches and staying energized naturally without having to resort to caffeine.

Servings: 1
Ingredients:
- Half cup of frozen or fresh blueberries
- 1 cup of fresh chopped spinach
- 1 cup of unsweetened almond milk or coconut milk
- 2 tablespoons of fresh chopped mint
- 1 teaspoon of stevia or a few banana slices

Optional (to garnish):

-a few mint leaves

-a slice of lime

Instructions:
1. Combine the spinach and almond milk in a high-speed blender.
2. Blend well until smooth and add the rest of the ingredients.
3. Blend again to make sure there are no lumps.
4. Pour your smoothie into a glass and enjoy right away.

Simple Raspberry Smoothie

Ever since I was a kid, I loved raspberries. It's one of my favourite fruits and whenever I can get it (I stick to seasonal options only) I turn them into smoothies. This one is miraculous and if you can combine it with some green powders you will create a nourishing green smoothie that is very tempting (great for green smoothie beginners). It's all about balance.

Serves: 1-2
Ingredients:
- 1 cup raspberries (you could also use blueberries)
- 1 cup almond milk or coconut milk
- Juice of 2 grapefruits
- Pinch of Himalayan salt
- Optional: 1 teaspoon of alfalfa or barley grass powder

Instructions:
1. Simply blend and serve.
2. Enjoy!

Refreshing Green Smoothie

Smoothies are always a great way to start your day and they are super quick to make. One smoothie a day will keep the doctor a way and it's better to schedule it first thing in the morning, before you get too busy.

Servings: 1 to 2
Ingredients:
- A few pineapple slices
- ½ cup baby spinach
- 1 cup coconut milk
- 6 to 8 ice cubes
- 1 teaspoon alfalfa powder or barley grass
- Juice of 2 limes

Instructions:
1. Combine the smoothie ingredients in a blender.
2. Blend until smooth and then add in the lime juice.
3. Pour your smoothie into a glass, drink and enjoy!

Sweet Cherry and Chia Smoothie

Servings: 1 to 2
Ingredients:
- ½ cup of frozen or fresh cherries
- ½ cup baby spinach
- 1 cup of almond milk
- 2 tablespoons of raw chia seeds
- Pinch ground ginger

Instructions:
1. Combine the smoothie ingredients in a blender.
2. First blend the spinach and cherries.
3. Add the milk, chia seeds and ginger.
4. Pour your finished smoothie into glasses and drink.

Spinach Green Tea Energy Smoothie

While caffeine in all its forms is not really alkaline, there is nothing wrong with an occasional cup of tea, especially green tea that is full of antioxidants and fat-burning properties. Great in a smoothie!

Servings: 2-3

Ingredients:
- 1 cup chopped baby spinach
- 1 small ripe avocado
- 1 cup brewed green tea, chilled
- Juice of 2 grapefruits
- Stevia to sweeten (optional)

Instructions:
1. Combine the smoothie ingredients in a blender and process a few times until smooth.
2. Pour your finished smoothie into glasses and drink.

Fruity Spicy Tropical Smoothie

While most fruit (especially "sugary" fruit) is not really alkaline, fruit is totally okay as a part of a balanced diet. It's also much healthier than processed carbs or sugary treats. There is no doubt about it. The spices used in this smoothie have anti-inflammatory and alkalizing properties and the green tea will give you a boost of energy.

Servings: 2-3
Ingredients:
- 1 cup blueberries
- 1 cup fresh papaya, chopped
- 1 medium banana
- A few ice cubes
- 2 cups brewed green tea, chilled
- 1 teaspoon ground turmeric
- 1 teaspoon ground ginger
- 1 teaspoon ground ginger
- Pinch cayenne pepper
- Optional: stevia

Instructions:
1. Combine the smoothie ingredients in a blender.
2. Blend well until smooth and add the spices.
3. Pour your finished smoothie into glasses and drink.
4. Enjoy!

Leafy Green Smoothie

Here is another smoothie that combines detoxifying and energizing properties. It is great to start your day feeling amazing!

Servings: 1 to 2
Ingredients:
- 1 cup of chopped kale
- 1 medium green apple, cored and chopped
- 1 stalk of celery, chopped
- ¼ cup of fresh parsley, minced
- 1 cup of fresh pomegranate or grapefruit juice
- A few ice cubes
- 1 tablespoon hemp seeds
- Stevia to sweeten (optional)

Instructions:
1. Combine the smoothie ingredients in a blender.
2. Blend well until smooth.
3. Pour your finished smoothie into a glass and drink.
4. Enjoy!

Super Alkalizing Avocado Coconut Smoothie

Servings: 1 to 2
Ingredients:
- 2 cups fresh chopped baby spinach
- 1 small chopped avocado
- ¼ cup of fresh chopped cilantro
- 1 cup chilled coconut water
- 1 tablespoon grated ginger, fresh
- ½ teaspoon ground turmeric
- Pinch cayenne

Instructions:
1. Combine the smoothie ingredients in your high-speed blender.
2. Pulse the ingredients a few times to chop them up.
3. Blend the mixture on the highest speed setting for 30 to 60 seconds.
4. Pour your finished smoothie into glasses and drink.
5. Enjoy!

Hydrating Watermelon Smoothie

This smoothie is great on a warm, summer morning, or anytime during the day. Watermelon combined with coconut water offer hydration, rejuvenation and energy.

Servings: 2-3
Ingredients:
- 1 cup frozen blueberries
- 1 cup fresh chopped watermelon
- 1 inch fresh sliced ginger
- 1 cup coconut water
- 1 tablespoon raw chia seeds
- A few ice cubes

Instructions:
1. Combine the smoothie ingredients in a blender.
2. Blend well until smooth.
3. Pour your finished smoothie into glasses and drink. Enjoy!

Ginger Protein Energy Smoothie

Servings: 1 to 2
Ingredients:
- 1 cup of chopped kale
- 1 cup pomegranates
- 1 medium carrot, diced
- 1 inch fresh grated ginger
- 1 cup coconut water
- 1 scoop hemp protein powder

Instructions:
1. Combine the smoothie ingredients in a blender.
2. Blend well until smooth.
3. Pour your finished smoothie into glasses and drink.

Peach Sweetness Smoothie

Servings: 1 to 2
Ingredients:
- 2 peaches, peeled and pitted
- 1 cup of almond milk
- 6 to 8 ice cubes
- 2 tablespoons raw hemp seeds or powder
- 1 teaspoon ground ginger
- Juice of 2 lemons

Instructions:
1. Combine the smoothie ingredients in a blender.
2. Blend until smooth, add ginger, ice cubes and hemp seeds.
3. Pour your finished smoothies into glasses and drink.
4. Enjoy!

Cucumber Melon Smoothie

I love this recipe in the summer! Honeydew melon gives it a nice taste which is great for those who are not used to drinking green smoothies.

Servings: 2
Ingredients:
- 1 cup of chopped honeydew melon
- 1 cup cucumber, diced
- 1 cup coconut water
- 1 tablespoon of fresh mint
- 1 tablespoon cilantro
- Pinch of Himalayan salt
- Juice of 1 lime
- Chia seeds (optional)

Instructions:
1. Blend the smoothie ingredients in a blender or food processor.
2. Add Himalayan salt to taste, mix well and if you wish, stir in some chia seeds for more nutrition.
3. Enjoy!

Fennel Magic Alka-Juice

Serves: 1-2
Ingredients:
- 2 cups fennel, chopped
- 2 tablespoons fennel seeds + 1 divided
- 2 cups spinach
- 2 cups carrot slices
- 1 pear, peeled and sliced
- ½ cup lemon juice
- Ice cubes

Instructions:

1. Wash all ingredients well. Clean and chop.
2. Add all ingredients (fennel, spinach, carrots, pear) through juicer.
3. Mix in some lemon juice. Place in a tall glass
4. Serve with a sprinkling of fennel seeds on top and it is best served chilled.
5. Ice cubes, and ginger ice cubes work great with this juice.
6. Enjoy!

Sweet Grapefruit Easy Mix

Pressed for time and want to alkalize? This recipe is super easy and full of alkalinity!

Serves: 1-2
Ingredients:

- 2 grapefruits
- 1 cup coconut water
- 1 cup almond milk
- ½ lemon
- 1 teaspoon powdered ginger
- ¼ cup warm water (not boiling)

Instructions:

1. Combine the powdered ginger and warm water until dissolved.
2. Add the lemon and grapefruit juice.
3. Add the coconut water and almond milk.
4. Add ice cubes or ginger ice cubes.
5. Enjoy!

Kukicha Smoothie

Ever heard of kukicha? If not, make sure you put it on your alkaline shopping list. If yes, I hope the following recipe will help you come up with more ideas on your alkaline journey!

Serves: 2
Ingredients:
- 1 cup kukicha tea
- 1 cup coconut milk
- ½ cup spinach
- 1 banana
- 1 inch ginger
- A green apple
- ¼ cup almonds (soaked in water for 8 hours or more)
- Optional: juice of 1 lemon

Instructions:
1. Blend all the ingredients until smooth.
2. For more alkalinity, add some lemon juice.
3. Stir well, serve, and enjoy!

Nice'n Fresh Smoothie

Soy sprouts and alfalfa sprouts are great, not only in your salads and soups, but also in your smoothies. When combined with other healthy and alkalizing ingredients, they create amazing alkaline balance and taste.

Serves: 2
Ingredients:
- 2 cups almond milk (unsweetened)
- ½ cup soy sprouts
- ½ cup alfalfa sprouts
- 1 inch ginger
- ½ an avocado
- 1 green apple
- 1 tablespoon avocado oil or coconut oil
- stevia to sweeten (optional)

Instructions:
1. Combine all the ingredients, except for oils, in a blender.
2. Blend until smooth.
3. Add some coconut oil or avocado oil. If you wish, sweeten with some stevia.
4. Enjoy!

Wake Up Maca Juice

Green, alkaline juices are natural energy boosters; however, by adding some maca powder, we can really take it to the next level!

Servings: 2-3
Ingredients:
- 1/2 cup water cress
- 3 big tomatoes
- A few fennel slices
- ½ inch ginger
- ½ cup parsley
- Juice of 1 lemon
- ½ teaspoon of maca powder
- 1 tablespoon olive oil or avocado oil

Procedure:
1. Wash and chop all the veggies.
2. Place through a juicer.
3. Place the juice in a tall glass and add some maca powder and lemon juice.
4. Add some olive or avocado oil for better absorption.

Additional Information:
Maca
This natural supplement is rich in Vitamin C, B, and E, as well as zinc, iron, calcium, magnesium, phosphorus, and amino acids. It has hormone balancing properties and acts as an aphrodisiac, both for men and women. As far as female health is concerned, maca can help alleviate menstrual cramps, as well as menopause issues (mood swings, depression, and anxiety).

Contraindications: avoid maca if pregnant or lactating. If on medication or suffering from any serious health problems, remember to contact your doctor first.

When trying maca for the first time, use no more than ½ teaspoon a day and go from there. The recommended maximum intake is actually about 1 teaspoon a day. However, remember that maca acts as a stimulant. Listen to your body; sometimes less is better.

Boost Your Metabolism Juice

This recipe offers a unique taste, pH balancing properties, metabolism boosting properties, and is also great for your skin.

Servings: 1-2
Ingredients:

- 1 cup fresh spinach
- 1 large grapefruit, juiced
- 1 carrot, small
- 2 celery stalks
- 1 beet
- ½ teaspoon cinnamon
- 1/2 inch of fresh stem ginger
- ¼ cup fresh mint leaves
- 1 tablespoon chia seeds

Procedure:

1. Wash the spinach, mint, grapefruit, carrot, celery stalks, and beet.
2. Chop the spinach, carrot (no need to peel if organic), celery, and beet.
3. Place through a juicer. While the juicer is working, you may juice the grapefruit (I use a simple lemon squeezer).
4. Mix the fresh veggie juice with grapefruit juice.
5. Add some chia seeds and stir well.
6. Drink immediately.
7. Enjoy!

Purple Energy Detox Juice

Beet root is extremely good for cleansing the liver. While I do agree it might not be the best juice for beginners, I can also tell you it's worth getting used to it. The juice is jam-packed with minerals and great for shedding unwanted pounds, not to mention higher energy levels! Lemon and lime juice add more flavor to this juice and make it a great, refreshing drink for any time of the day.

Servings: 1-2
Ingredients:
- 2 celery stalks
- 2 medium cucumbers
- ¼ cup parsley
- ¼ cup mint
- 1 beet root
- 1 lemon, juiced
- 1 lime, juiced
- 1 tsp olive oil
- Pinch of Himalayan salt

Procedure:
1. Wash and chop all the ingredients.
2. Place celery, cucumbers, parsley, mint and beet root through a juicer.
3. When ready, place the juice in a juice glass or another utensil of your choice and stir in some lemon and lime juice, as well as Himalayan salt and a bit of olive oil (or any other quality cold-pressed oil) of your choice. Oils help your body with nutrient absorption. Enjoy!

SECTION III Hunger Satisfying Alkaline Recipes

Chilled Spicy Avocado Soup

I know what you are thinking... "Soup... for breakfast?" Well, everything is possible in the alkaline world. This recipe is perfect if you want to increase your energy levels; it's raw and 100% alkaline! You can even prepare more and save it in your fridge to have a healthy, energizing elixir to sip on during the day. It's a great recipe if you wish to reduce inflammation, detoxify and start losing weight.

Servings: 2
Ingredients:
- 2 large avocados, pitted and chopped
- 2 cucumbers, peeled and diced
- 1/2 cup coconut yogurt or coconut cream
- 2 tablespoons of chopped chives
- 2 tablespoons of cilantro
- 1 tablespoon of fresh lime juice
- 1 teaspoon of Himalayan salt
- ½ small jalapeno, seeded and minced
- Pinch of cayenne pepper or black pepper to taste (curry is also an option)
- 1 teaspoon of minced ginger
- 1/2 teaspoon of minced garlic

Instructions:
1. Place all the ingredients (except spices) in a food processor and blend until smooth.
2. Add chives, cilantro, lime juice. Himalaya salt, jalapeno, pepper, ginger and garlic
3. You can add in some water if you don't like thick consistency.
4. Pour the soup into a serving bowl and chill it for at least an hour until cold.
5. Another option is to have this soup slightly warm.
6. Enjoy!

Thai Tofu and Vegetable Curry

I know what you're thinking, "Curry for breakfast?" Well, why not? It's a great option if you wake up hungry or are looking for a filling breakfast recipe after a morning workout. This recipe is fantastic on a cold, winter morning and relatively quick to make.

Servings: 2

Ingredients:
- 1 cup of vegetable broth (low sodium)
- 1 cup of coconut milk
- ½ tablespoon of Thai red curry paste
- ¼ teaspoon ground ginger
- Himalayan salt to taste
- 1 cup red bell pepper
- Half cup green beans, trimmed
- 1 cup of chopped carrots
- 1 medium sweet potato, peeled and chopped
- ½ cup of diced tofu
- 1 tablespoon of fresh lime juice
- 1 tablespoons of fresh chopped basil

Instructions:
1. Combine the vegetable broth, coconut milk, ginger and salt and curry paste in a medium saucepan.
2. Bring to a boil.
3. Stir in red bell pepper, beans, carrots and sweet potato.
4. Simmer for 5 minutes until just turning tender.
5. Stir in the tofu and cook for a few minutes more.
6. Finally, add in some lime juice, basil, salt and pepper to taste.
7. Serve hot. Enjoy!

Breakfast Kale Soup

I know that many people can be put off by the name of this recipe, but don't reject it before you have tried it. Kale is miraculous and this soup will help keep you warm and energized on cold winter mornings. It can also be served chilled as a natural tool to feed your body with nutrients.

Serves: 2
Ingredients:
1 small onion, chopped
3 cloves garlic, minced
2 celery stalks, diced
2 tablespoons red wine
4 tablespoons olive oil or coconut oil
4 cups vegetable stock
1 teaspoon Himalayan salt
¼ teaspoon black pepper
¼ teaspoon dried basil (or 1 tsp fresh)
1 can cooked chickpeas, rinsed and drained
1 cup kale no stems, ale, cut into strips

Instructions:
1. First, sauté celery, garlic and onion in the oil for 3-4 minutes (medium heat)
2. Add veggie stock as well as basil, chickpeas, salt and pepper.
3. Bring to a boil (covered).
4. Reduce heat and simmer for about 15 minutes on medium heat.
5. Blend the mixture.
6. Once blended, pour the mixture back into the pot, adding the kale and simmering for 10 minutes.
7. Serve hot.
8. Enjoy!

Awesome Alkaline Tacos

Great breakfast idea if you wake up feeling hungry or are not in the mood for smoothies or porridges.

Serves: 2-4
Ingredients:
- 4 gluten-free tortillas
- 1 cooked sweet potato
- Green beans
- Salad greens (kale, spinach, lettuce, chard, arugula - it's up to you)
- 1 avocado, peeled, pitted and sliced
- Half cup black beans, cooked
- Spices to taste (cumin, chili powder, garlic powder, onion powder and cayenne pepper are my favorite)

Instructions:
1. If you wish, warm the tortillas in the oven or over the stove. Careful not to burn them. I suggest you heat them on a low flame for 10 seconds on each side.
2. Blend the sweet potato with the spices.
3. Spread the mixture across the center of each tortilla. Add beans, avocado and greens on top.
4. Serve with some fresh tomato and tomato slices for more alkaline properties.
5. Enjoy!

Energizing Breakfast Potatoes Brunch

This is a fantastic brunch recipe for those who are starving!

Serves: 2
Ingredients:
- 2 tablespoons olive oil
- 2 cups sweet potatoes
- 1 large onion
- 2 tablespoons capers
- Vegan sour cream
- 1 Tablespoon Dijon mustard
- Salt and pepper to taste
- Mixed greens for side salad

Instructions:
1. Wash, peel and chop potatoes.
2. Take a medium-size skillet and heat up the olive oil, adding potatoes and scallions (medium-heat)
3. Sautee adding some water until potatoes are soft. Keep stirring.
4. Combine all remaining ingredients in a bowl, except the greens. Place on a plate and pour sour cream mixture on top.
5. Serve with green leafy greens.
6. Enjoy!

Red Pepper Hummus

This hummus is great with some raw veggies, gluten free wraps or homemade bread!

Servings: 10 to 12

Ingredients:
- 1.5 cup chickpeas, cooked, rinsed and drained
- 1 cup of roasted red peppers, chopped
- 2 cloves minced garlic
- 1/4 jalapeno, seeded and minced
- Himalayan salt and black pepper to taste
- 4 tablespoons olive oil
- Water, as needed

Instructions:
1. Combine the chickpeas, roasted red pepper, garlic and jalapeno in a food processor.
2. Blend well until smooth.
3. Season with salt and pepper to taste.
4. Add in the oil and water for desired consistency.
5. Serve with sliced veggies, in wraps and sandwiches.
6. Enjoy!

Baked Spicy Kale Chips

Servings: 4 to 6
Ingredients:
- 3 cups of kale leaves
- Olive oil or coconut oil
- Himalayan salt, black pepper, curry powder (or your favourite spices), to taste

Instructions:
1. Preheat the oven to 220°F and line two rimmed baking sheets with parchment paper.
2. Massage the kale leaves in oil and spread them on baking sheets in a single layer.
3. Sprinkle liberally with spices and add salt.
4. Bake for 40 minutes, carefully flipping the sides. Kale is easy to burn to keep an eye on the oven.
5. Turn off the oven and let the kale cool until crisp.
6. Enjoy!
7. Serve with hummus or vegetable dips. You can also take it as a take away breakfast or snack.

Simple Bean Breakfast
Quick and Easy!

Serves: 2
Ingredients:
- 1 can white haricot beans
- 4 spring onions (early picked, red onion) chopped
- 6 grape tomatoes halved or quartered
- 2 tablespoons fresh chopped basil
- 2 cups fresh spinach
- 3 cloves chopped garlic
- 1 avocado (peeled and pitted)
- ½ squeezed lemon
- Coconut/olive oil
- Himalayan salt/black pepper
- Leafy greens (side salad) of your choice - enough for 2 people

Preparation:
1. Heat about 3 tablespoons water in a frying pan and steam fry chopped garlic (about one minutes.).
2. Add tomatoes, beans and onions, until soft.
3. Put in the basil and spinach. Allow to wilt, and then sprinkle with pepper and salt.
4. Slice the avocado. Put the bean mix over the greens and top with avocado. Drizzle olive oil over the top and finish with a squeeze of lemon.
5. Enjoy!

Alkaline Green Wraps

Do you know the feeling when you wake up hungry? Well, the alkaline solution is simple - go for alkaline, gluten free wraps!

Serves: 1
Ingredients:
- 2 gluten-free, yeast-free wraps
- 1 cup of radish, chopped
- 2 garlic cloves, chopped
- ½ cup of freshly made hummus or tahini
- 1 avocado, sliced
- 1 cucumber, peeled and diced

Preparation (2 simple steps for busy people!)
1. Mix all the ingredients in a salad bowl. Add olive oil, lemon juice, tahini (or hummus) and Himalayan salt.
2. Place the filling in each wrap, roll up and serve!
3. Enjoy! Alkaline wraps are real life savers. They keep you full, alkalize your body and mind, and you don't feel like you are missing something...

Raw Alkaline Breakfast

Have you ever considered having delicious alkaline salads first thing in the morning? If not, why not? This recipe is great for hot summers! Raw foods and alkalinity go hand in hand!

Serves: 1
Ingredients:

- Half avocado
- ½ cup of alfalfa sprouts
- 2 tomatoes
- 1 cucumber
- 2 onion rings, minced
- Half garlic clove, minced
- 1 tablespoon avocado oil
- ¼ cup of raw almonds
- Himalayan salt and black pepper to taste
- Optional: ¼ cup cooked lentils or chickpeas (great in the winter)
- Juice of half a lemon

Preparation:

1. Mix all the veggies in a salad bowl.
2. Drizzle over some avocado oil, lemon juice and season with Himalayan salt and black pepper.
3. Enjoy!

SECTION IV

Alkaline Paleo Recipes

The recipes from this section are a blend of a paleo and alkaline diet. They offer a variety of grain-free and alkalizing meals that are also paleo friendly and most of them are vegetarian friendly. I believe that the paleo diet is not only about eating massive amounts of meat. It's all about balance and variety. The following recipes are great for alkaline diet beginners or those who need to take small baby steps to make a transition and can't imagine jumping into the green smoothies or raw foods all at once. Remember to listen to your body; it never lies!

Paleo Tomato Basil Omelet (Vegetarian)

Eggs are far from alkalizing, but we can balance them with greens, vegetables and spices to obtain a highly nutritious and balanced meal. Great for beginners!

Servings: 1
Ingredients:
- 2 teaspoons coconut oil
- 1 medium ripe tomato, chopped
- 2 tablespoons sweet onion, chopped
- Himalayan Salt and black pepper to taste
- 2 organic eggs, whisked well
- 1 tablespoon fresh chopped chives
- A handful of fresh basil leaves, chopped
- ¼ cup spinach and arugula leaves, mixed

Instructions:
1. Heat coconut oil in a small non-stick skillet.
2. Switch to medium heat, add the tomato and onion seasoning with salt and pepper.
3. Cook for a couple of minutes until the onion is translucent then transfer into a small bowl.

4. Reheat the skillet using the same remaining oil.
5. In the meantime, beat the egg with the chives.
6. Transfer the mixture into the skillet and season with salt and pepper.
7. Let the egg cook for about 1 minute then swirl the pan to spread the uncooked egg.
8. Cook for another minute or two until the egg is almost set.
9. Placed the cooked vegetables over the omelette (just one side) and sprinkle with basil.
10. Then fold the empty half of the omelette over the fillings.
11. Cook for 1 minute or until the egg is set – slide onto a plate and serve hot with some spinach and arugula leaves on side.
12. Enjoy!

Banana Coffee Bread (Vegetarían, Paleo)

While this is not a super alkaline recipe, it's all natural and full of anti-inflammatory properties. We already know that balance is the key, and the alkaline diet is not only about eating 100% alkaline, we need variety. This version is made with natural sweeteners and gluten free flour. It is much lower in carbohydrates than an average processed cake. While it's not something I recommend you have every day, it's great as a weekend treat. Imagine starting your day with banana bread and a nice cup of herbal tea! Something to look forward to.

Serves: 6
Ingredients:
- 3 brown bananas, mashed
- 1 teaspoon vanilla extract
- Liquid stevia to sweeten (optional)
- 3 eggs
- ½ cup almond butter
- ¼ cup coconut flour
- ½ teaspoon baking soda
- ½ teaspoon baking powder
- 1 teaspoon cinnamon
- pinch of Himalayan salt

For the toppings
- 4 tablespoons coconut oil
- 2 tablespoons almond flour
- 1 teaspoon cinnamon
- ¼ cup pecans, crushed

Instructions:
1. First, grease your baking dish with oil lining with parchment paper.
2. In a bowl, mix together almond butter, eggs, vanilla, stevia, and bananas.
3. Add baking powder, baking soda, coconut flour, cinnamon and salt.
4. Mix well together.

5. Pour the batter into a baking dish and place on a baking sheet.
6. In a second bowl, add coconut oil, almond flour, cinnamon, coconut sugar and pecans.
7. Mix all toppings together using your hands.
8. Place chunks of toppings on top of the banana bread mixture. Spread evenly. Bake for 50 minutes.
9. Remove, cool for about 20 minutes and serve.
10. Enjoy!

Spinach Frittata

We all know spinach is good for us, but few people actually enjoy it. Well, if you wish to add more greens into your diet and change your relationship with spinach, this is a recipe for you.

Servings: 3-4
Ingredients:
- 2 tablespoons coconut oil
- Half cup green pepper, sliced
- 1 medium red bell pepper, sliced
- 1 clove garlic, minced
- Himalayan salt and pepper to taste
- ¼ cup baby spinach, chopped
- 3 large eggs, whisked well
- 1 tablespoon unsweetened almond milk
- ¼ cup fresh arugula leaves or and basil leaves
- Half avocado per serving

Instructions:

1. Using a medium skillet, heat the coconut oil on the medium-high heat.
2. Add the red and green bell pepper and garlic, adding in salt and pepper.
3. Cook for a couple of minutes and add in the spinach.
4. Let the spinach cook for 1 minute (until slightly wilted) then remove from the heat.
5. Take a mixing bowl and beat together the almond milk, eggs, pinch of salt and pepper to taste.
6. Stir in the spinach and pepper mixture.
7. Reheat the skillet on the medium heat setting until very hot.
8. Pour in the egg and vegetable mixture and swirl the pan to spread the mixture evenly.
9. Cook for a few minutes, stirring occasionally, until the eggs along the bottom of are set.
10. Serve with arugula leaves and half avocado on side.

Alkaline Paleo Zucchini/Sweet Potato Pancakes (Vegetarian)

This recipe is very easy to make and an excellent start of the day!

It's like traditional Spanish "tortilla de patata" or "tortilla de calabazin", but much healthier as it is served with alkalizing veggies instead of a white processed baguette.

Serves: 2
Ingredients:
- 3 eggs
- 1 tbsp. coconut flour
- Himalayan salt and black pepper to taste
- 2 cups shredded zucchini, or sweet potato
- Coconut oil
- 1 avocado (half per serving), peeled, pitted, sliced
- Half cup radish, sliced
- 1 tomato (half per serving), sliced
- 1 big cucumber (half per serving), sliced or spiralized
- Olive oil

Instructions:
1. Beat eggs with coconut flour adding pepper and Himalayan salt.
2. Place sweet potato or zucchini through a food processor until smooth.
3. Mix in the zucchini or sweet potato mix with the eggs until well combined.
4. Add coconut oil to the skillet (medium heat).
5. Form sweet potato (or zucchini) batter into pancakes of your size and cook on the skillet until done, about 2-3 minutes per side.
6. Switch off the heat and let it cool down.
7. In the meantime, take a small salad bowl and combine avocado, cucumber, tomato and radish. Toss well adding some olive oil and Himalayan salt to taste.
8. Serve your pancakes with the fresh, alkaline salad.
9. Enjoy!

Alkaline Paleo Coconut Muffins (Vegetarian)

This recipe is great for beginners and it makes muffin creation super easy.

Serves: 2
Ingredients:

- 1/4 cup + 1 tbsp. coconut flour
- 3 eggs
- 2 tablespoon melted coconut oil
- 1/4 cup whole coconut milk
- 1/4 tsp baking powder
- Cinnamon and nutmeg to taste
- Pinch of Himalayan salt

Instructions:

1. Pre-heat oven to 400 °F (200°C)
2. Mix all ingredients energetically, make sure there are no lumps.
3. Pour into greased or lined muffin tin.
4. Bake for about 12-15 minutes.
5. Serve with some fresh alkaline fruit, like for example grapefruits (great for Vitamin C and energy first thing in the morning)
6. You can always store your muffins in a freezer and reheat later.
7. Enjoy!

Alkaline Paleo Breakfast Mix

This is how we can easily add more greens into our diets...

Serves: 2-4
Ingredients:
- 2 tablespoons coconut oil (melted)
- 1 large sweet potato or yam, diced
- ½ teaspoon Himalayan salt
- A few salmon slices (one per serving)
- ½ onion, diced
- 2 cups spinach, finely chopped
- 5 eggs, whisked
- ½ teaspoon Himalayan salt
- A teaspoon garlic powder

Instructions:
1. First, grease a 9 x 12 baking sheet and preheat oven to 400 °F (200°C).
2. Toss diced sweet potatoes in coconut oil and top with Himalayan salt.
3. Place potatoes in baking sheet and bake until soft, about 20 minutes.
4. In the meantime, place a sauté pan over medium heat, adding onion and salmon. Cook until salmon is done.
5. Place salmon and onion mixture into the baking dish, adding sweet potatoes, spinach and eggs. Sprinkle over some Himalayan salt and garlic powder and mix well until well combined.
6. Bake for about 15 minutes, until eggs are fully cooked.
7. Serve with greens like spinach or arugula or avocado on side.
8. Enjoy!

Nori Hand-roll Mix

If you are crazy about sushi, you will love this recipe. Nori is full of macronutrients and is also a great component of salads and soups. But of course, it's mostly famous as a sushi component.

Ingredients:
- 1 toasted nori seaweed sheet
- 1 small avocado, mashed
- Half cup smoked salmon chunks
- A few slices of cucumber
- 1 green onion finely chopped
- Lemon (optional)

Instructions:
1. Place nori sheet on a cutting board.
2. Add the avocado, salmon, cucumber, and onion, top with lemon if desired. Wrap it up and enjoy! It's also great as brunch/lunch or even as a snack.

Energizing Matcha Crepes (Paleo, Vegetarian)

Looking for an easy way to reduce your intake of or stop drinking coffee? Try some matcha crepes! Nothing feel better than homemade gluten free food.

Servings: 10 to 12
Ingredients:
- 1 ¼ cups almond flour
- 1 to 2 teaspoons matcha powder
- 2 large eggs, beaten well
- 1 cup of almond milk
- 2 tablespoons of coconut oil, melted
- A few drops of stevia
- 1 teaspoon of vanilla extract
- 1 teaspoon cinnamon powder

Instructions:
1. Combine all of the ingredients in a blender.
2. Blend well until smooth.
3. Heat a small non-stick skillet on the low heat and spray with cooking spray.
4. Pour in about ¼ cup of batter and tilt the pan to evenly coat the bottom.
5. Cook for a couple of minutes until the edges of the crepe are dry and browned.
6. Flip the side and cook for another 1 minute or so until the crepe is fully cooked and then transfer them to a plate to keep warm.
7. Repeat the process to make more crepes.
8. Serve with fresh alkaline fruits, like pomegranate or grapefruits.
9. Enjoy!

Easy Veggie Alkaline Paleo Bake (Vegetarian)

Servings: 5
Ingredients:
- 1 tablespoon coconut oil
- 1 cup diced green pepper
- 1 cup diced sweet potato
- 1 cup chopped zucchini
- 1 onion, chopped
- 2 cups fresh chopped spinach
- 5 large eggs, beaten well
- Himalayan salt and pepper to taste

Instructions:
1. Preheat the oven to 375°F and grease your baking dish with coconut oil.
2. In the meantime, prepare a large skillet on the medium heat and heat up some coconut oil.
3. Add the sweet potatoes, zucchini and onion – cook for 8 to 10 minutes until tender.
4. Stir in the spinach and cook for 1 to 2 minutes.
5. Transfer the veggies into the baking dish.
6. Beat the eggs with the salt and pepper then pour into the dish as well. Mix well.
7. Bake for 25 to 30 minutes until the center is set.
8. Allow the casserole to cool for 10 minutes before serving.
9. Enjoy!

Breakfast Zucchini Pasta with Salmon

This recipe is just great if you get up feeling hungry or are looking for a quick brunch recipe!

Serves: 1
Ingredients:
- 1 zucchini, spiralized
- 2 slices of smoked salmon
- 2 tablespoons coconut oil
- Black pepper
- Himalayan salt
- Garlic powder

To serve:
- Half avocado (sprinkled with lime or lemon juice and pinch of Himalayan salt)
- Cilantro
- Cucumber slices

Instructions:
1. Heat up some coconut oil in a pan (medium heat).
2. Add the spiralized zucchini with a pinch of Himalayan salt, black pepper and garlic powder.
3. Cook until zucchini gets soft using low heat.
4. Then add salmon slices and stir well. Keep cooking for a couple of minutes more.
5. Serve with avocado, cilantro and cucumber slices.
6. Enjoy!

Afterword- Stay Alkaline and Don't Worry Too Much!

The aim of this recipe book was to show you how you can adapt to a clean alkaline diet. This alkaline inspired cuisine allows you to still eat mouth-watering, healthy, wholesome meals that will enable you to live life to the fullest without feeling deprived.

I really hope you'll continue to get a lot of use out of this book as you progress with your alkaline diet lifestyle returning again and again to your favourite recipes. Here's wishing you all the best in your health and wellness journey!

For more inspiration and empowerment, please meet me at: www.HolisticWellnessProject.com

I wish you wellness and energy,

Marta Tuchowska

Book2
The Alkaline Diet Lifestyle Cookbook
Vol.2

Delectable Alkaline Lunch Recipes for Vibrant Health, Unstoppable Energy, and Massive Weight Loss

By Marta Tuchowska (aka Marta Wellness)
Copyright ©Marta Tuchowska 2015

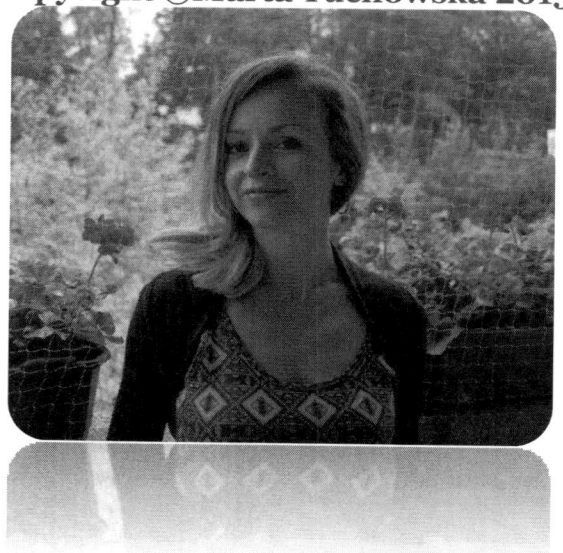

www.HolisticWellnessProject.com
www.amazon.com/author/mtuchowska

IMPORTANT

The book is not intended to provide medical advice or to take the place of medical advice and treatment from your personal physician. Readers are advised to consult their own doctors or other qualified health professionals regarding the treatment of medical conditions. The author shall not be held liable or responsible for any misunderstanding or misuse of the information contained in this book. The information is not intended to diagnose, treat or cure any disease.

It is important to remember that the author of this book is not a doctor/ medical professional. Only opinions based upon her own personal experiences or research are cited. THE AUTHOR DOES NOT OFFER MEDICAL ADVICE or prescribe any treatments. For any health or medical issues – you should be talking to your doctor first.

Amazing Alkaline Lunches

It's quite easy to make an alkaline, vegan-style lunch when you're inspired by the massive range of delicious plant-based items you can choose from. The problem, though, is not getting stuck in a rut and eating the same old salad, day in day out. This selection of delicious recipes aims to avoid precisely that. Mix your lunchtime up a little and try one of these tasty and nutritious lunch dishes.

Warning: eating more alkaline will make you more energized. Your skin will glow. You will feel happier and more focused, and you will be less prone to colds and flu, and (if desired) you will start losing weight. Your friends will keep asking you - what have you been doing? So, if you are not ready for the above mentioned benefits, refrain from eating a healthy alkaline-inspired diet and don't even try my recipes!

Alkaline Variety Mix
Taco Salad

In any diet (alkaline or not), it is extremely important to sneak in some raw vegetables for more energy and health. The alkaline diet and raw foods go hand in hand and you can easily combine both. Let's have a look at nutrition: sunflower seeds are great in salads, smoothies or even as a snack. They are high in vitamin E and copper, and even offer some protein. On top of that, you will nourish your body with plenty of vitamins and minerals from the veggies as well as good fats from the avocado.

Serves: 2-3
Ingredients:
Sunflower "Vegan Meat":
- 2/3 cup sunflower seeds (preferably soaked in water for a few hours)
- 1 tsp. chili powder

- 1 tsp. cumin
- ½ tsp. cayenne pepper
- Himalayan salt to taste

Cashew Cream Salsa:
- 1 cup cashew nuts, soaked for a few hours (you can also use almonds instead of cashews, almonds are much more alkaline-forming, but to be honest I am addicted to cashews)
- 1 cup water (feel free to experiment with thickness)
- juice of 1 fresh lime + juice of half a lemon
- Himalayan salt to taste
- Black pepper to taste (optional)
- Half teaspoon maca powder for energy (optional)

Super Alkaline Guacamole:
- 1 avocado, peeled, chopped, pitted
- 1/4 cup onion, chopped
- 2 tomatoes, chopped
- ½ tsp. cumin
- juice of 1 fresh lemon or lime
- Himalayan salt to taste
- 1 tablespoon olive oil

Salad:
2 cups mixed greens of your choice (recommend baby spinach, parsley, dill, cilantro and arugula- yum!)

Instructions:
1. Place all the "vegan meat" ingredients through a blender or food processor. Add spices. Mix well.
2. Get ready for the cashew sauce. Place some soaked cashews (or almonds) in a blender adding water and lemon/lime juice. Blend until smooth. Add salt, pepper and maca powder for more energy (careful though- maca is an aphrodisiac)
3. Now, blend all the guacamole ingredients together. Mix well.

4. Now, it's time to take care of the salad. First, prepare some salad bowls and add your greens. Place guacamole on top. Then, add cashew salsa and vegan meat on top.
5. Enjoy!

Vegan Chili

I love this recipe on cold winter days. It combines two types of highly nutritional beans which are essential for fiber and protein. Spices have anti-inflammatory properties and add an amazing, oriental flavour. The recipe is also great for busy folks, as you can do some serious batch-coking and then simply take this for lunches and dinners to save your precious time. Organization and planning are key to success.

Serves: 3-4
Ingredients:
- 4 tbsp. extra virgin olive oil (or coconut oil)
- 1 cup diced onion (preferably red)
- 5 cloves garlic, minced
- 2 jalapeno peppers, diced
- 2 green bell pepper, finely chopped
- 1 cup celery, finely chopped
- 1 cup diced tomatoes
- 3 cups vegetable broth
- ¼ cup tomato paste
- ½ cup kidney beans, cooked
- ½ cup pinto beans, cooked
- 1 tsp. cumin
- 1 tsp. chili powder
- 2 tsps. oregano
- 1 tsp. cayenne pepper (optional)
- Himalayan salt and pepper to taste

Optional:
Choose your favorite chili toppings, such as vegan sour cream or fresh cilantro.

Instructions:
1. In a large soup pot, heat some oil using medium heat. Then, add onion and garlic. Stir well until onion is soft.
2. Add a few pinches of Himalayan salt and keep stirring.
3. Add jalapenos bell pepper and celery. Stir all together for a few minutes.

4. Add diced tomatoes, veggie broth, and tomato paste.
5. Stirring well until combined.
6. Then, add pinto and kidney beans along with all other spices (chili, cumin, oregano, cayenne and salt). Simmer until your chili becomes thick, for roughly 15 minutes.
7. Serve with toppings of your choice.

OPTIONAL: if you are looking for more energy, you could add some quinoa, brown rice or sweet potato.

Amazingly Alkaline Avocado Chickpea Salad

This is a fantastic recipe I learned from a vegan body builder friend of mine and remodified it slightly to make it more alkaline. The more I learn about veganism and vegan body builders and their ways of eating the more inspired I get. Meat is not the only way to get protein, there are so many other, more sustainable plant-based sources of protein available. Of course, the choice is yours. Nothing is set in stone so feel free to personalize my recipes. Now, let's have a look at the simple nutritional side of things: Garbanzo beans are high in fiber, which is essential for healthy digestion, and avocadoes are rich in good fats, which are vital for cell maintenance and function. It's like healthy fat that can help us burn bad fat!

Serves: 2-4
Ingredients:
- 1 cup chickpeas, cooked
- 1 cup baby spinach
- 1 avocado, peeled, pitted, cubed
- 1/4 cup fresh cilantro leaves, chopped
- ½ white onion, thinly sliced
- 2 zucchini, spiralized or sliced super thin
- juice of 1 fresh lemon + 1 lime
- 2 tbsp. coconut oil
- Himalayan salt and black pepper to taste
- 2 tsps. curry powder
- A handful or raisins
- 2 tablespoons chia seeds

Instructions:
1. Heat up some coconut oil in a pan (medium heat).
2. Gently stir-fry spiralized zucchinis adding curry powder and Himalayan salt.
3. When slightly soft, add chickpeas and keep stir-frying for a few minutes.
4. Remove from heat and let it cool down.

5. In the meantime, prepare the salad: combine avocado, cilantro, onion and baby spinach in a salad bowl. Toss well.
6. Now add the spiralized zucchinis and chickpeas. Sprinkle over some lime or lemon juice. Add chia seeds and raisins.
7. Season with Himalayan salt if necessary.
8. Enjoy!

Vegan Energy Bowl

If you are looking for a massive variety of important macro and micro nutrients as well as amazing taste, this recipe is your next stop. Moreover, it proves that healthy eating can be done on a budget and even on a busy schedule (check out the additional resource after the end of this recipe for more tips). Let's have a look at some of the nutritional benefits: Red cabbage is high in vitamin K (great for bone health) and vitamin C (immune system health). Sweet potatoes are a great source of natural, unprocessed carbs (have no fear) and are also high in vitamin C. Add to it protein from the beans and alkalizing benefits of dark leafy greens. Healthy, delicious, easy and hunger satisfying. Great for active lifestyles.

Serves: 2-4
Ingredients:

- 2 sweet potatoes, washed and cubed
- 1 cup black beans, cooked and drained
- 1 cup brown rice or quinoa
- 2 carrots, sliced
- 2 beets, sliced
- ¼ purple cabbage, shredded
- 2 cups kale or other greens like spinach, Swiss chard, or similar
- juice of 1 fresh lemon
- 2 avocados, sliced
- hummus of your choice (zucchinis or chickpea)
- 2 tbsps. coconut oil
- Himalayan salt and pepper to taste

Instructions:

1. Preheat oven to 400 degrees Fahrenheit (about 200 degrees Celsius).
2. In the meantime, peel and dice the potatoes.
3. Smear some coconut oil over the baking dish and place your sweet potato cubes in it.
4. Add some salt and pepper to taste and begin baking.

5. Bake for about 30 minutes so that sweet potato gets tender.
6. In the meantime, you can prepare your quinoa or brown rice. (I usually cook quinoa in batches and I always have some cooked quinoa in my fridge which makes recipes faster and easier.)
7. Now, it's time for some creative plate arrangements so that we can eat mindfully and peacefully. Feel free to use your imagination and...
8. Place roasted sweet potato, chickpeas, rice/other grain on the plate(s). Add carrots, cabbage, greens, hummus and avocado bites.
9. Season with lemon or lime juice, Himalayan salt and other spices of your choice,
10. Let the alkaline vegan feast begin!

Additional resources to read or listen to (article blog post + audio post):
Healthy Eating on a Busy Schedule
www.holisticwellnessproject.com/blog/alkaline-diet/alkaline-lifestyle-for-busy-people/
Mindful Eating
www.holisticwellnessproject.com/blog/mindfulness/mindful-eating/

Easy Alkaline Sandwich

I used to think that going alkaline meant no more sandwiches. I was wrong! It all comes down to choosing the right bread (the more natural the better and gluten-free is always more recommended on an alkaline diet). The following sandwich recipe treats us with all the health benefit of fresh basil (high in vitamin K and has cell protective flavonoids). Moreover, it will leave you feeling satisfied and nicely energized, keep your belly happy and is full of protein. It makes an excellent take away lunch as well.

Serves: 1
Ingredients
Alkaline Pesto:
- 1/2 cup fresh basil
- ¼ cup cilantro leaves
- 1/3 cup walnuts
- 1 garlic clove
- 2 tablespoons extra virgin olive oil
- juice of 1 fresh lemon
- Himalayan salt and pepper to taste

Sandwich:
- 2 slices multi-grain or sprouted-grain bread (gluten free, if sensitive)
- 2 tbsp. home- made hummus or tahini
- 2 tbsp. pesto
- 1 small tomato, sliced
- ½ avocado, sliced
- Lettuce, spinach or other greens of your choice (optional)

Instructions:
1. First prepare the pesto: place all the pesto ingredients (except olive oil) in a blender or food processor. Add some olive oil to achieve the desired consistency (I prefer to keep it thick).

2. Prepare the sandwich- you can toast the bread slices if you wish. Then, spread hummus and pesto on the slices.
3. Add avocado slices, tomato slices, and other greens of your choice.
4. Enjoy!

Alkalizing Coco Gazpacho-Inspired Soup

Tomatoes offer an antioxidant called lycopene, which studies show to be strongly tied to bone health. Moreover, they help us rehydrate and alkalize. While the traditional Spanish gazpacho is a recipe usually associated with hot summers (it was originally created in Andalucía- the Southern province of Spanish, where it gets extremely hot in the summer), you can actually have it all year long. You can always personalize it by adding some nuts, seeds, quinoa, red lentils etc.

Serves: 2-4
Ingredients:
- 4 large tomatoes, peeled and chopped
- 3 cucumbers, peeled and chopped
- 1 red bell pepper, chopped
- 1 onion, finely chopped
- 1 cup coconut milk (raw, unsweetened)
- ½ cup alkaline water
- 2 tbsp. fresh cilantro leaves
- 3 cloves garlic, peeled and minced
- Juice of 1 lemon
- Himalayan Salt and pepper to taste
- 2 tbsps. olive oil
- Cayenne pepper to taste
- Tabasco to taste (optional)

Instructions:
1. Place all the ingredients through a blender (except olive oil and spices).
2. Blend well and add olive oil, salt and spices.
3. Stir well.
4. You can serve it cool, as the original Spanish recipe recommends, or slightly warm.
5. Feel free to make it spicier with tabasco.
6. Enjoy!

Black Beans and Basmati Rice (serves 4-6)

Here's a dish that can help you get plenty of good quality protein and a decent helping of fiber all at once. Avocado and lime (as well as tomatoes) add to alkalizing properties of this balanced vegan lunch.

Ingredients:
- 2 tbsp. olive oil
- 1 medium onion, chopped
- 1 large red bell pepper, deseeded and chopped
- 1 clove of garlic, chopped
- 2 medium tomatoes, chopped
- 1 cup cooked black beans
- 3/4 cup raw basmati rice, well rinsed
- 2 cups water
- Himalayan salt and black pepper to taste
- Half avocado for each serving
- 1 lime
- 1 tablespoon fresh cilantro for each serving

Instructions:
1. Add the olive oil to a large saucepan placed over a medium heat. Sauté the onion and bell pepper until the onion becomes translucent in appearance.
2. Add the garlic and tomatoes to the saucepan and season to taste with the salt and black pepper.
3. Cook this mixture for a couple of minutes and then add the black beans and rice.
4. Add the water and stir the mixture well.
5. Bring the mixture to the boil and then cover the saucepan with the lid.
6. Reduce to a simmer and cook for 15-25 minutes, until the water has been absorbed.
7. Use a fork to fluff the mixture up and then serve with avocado halves. Sprinkle over some lime juice, Himalayan salt and cilantro on top of avocado.
8. Enjoy!

Roasted Coconut Eggplant

It's important to find a healthy source of plant fats when following the alkaline way, so what better than to use eggplant to soak up the delicious flavors of fresh coconut milk!

Servings: 4
Ingredients:
- 1 large eggplant, sliced into 1/4 inch thick circles
- 1 large onion, chopped
- 1 fresh chili pepper or 1 tsp. dried chili flakes (optional)
- 1.75 cup of coconut milk
- Salt and black pepper to taste

Instructions
1. Preheat the oven to 350 degrees Fahrenheit (175 Celsius).
2. Set out a layer of eggplant slices in a large casserole dish.
3. Layer some of the onion over the top of the eggplant, and then add some chili, salt and pepper to taste.
4. Repeat these layers until you have two or three layers. Then pour the coconut milk over the top.
5. Cover the casserole dish with aluminium foil to seal everything in.
6. Bake in the oven for 45-60 minutes, until the eggplant becomes soft.
7. Remove the foil and bake for another 10 minutes to allow the liquid to reduce.
8. Serve while still hot, or allow to cool slightly.
9. Enjoy!

Comforting Carrot Ginger

Ginger root is miraculous and has a whole range of anti-inflammatory properties. This recipe is great as digestive tonic and it also helps prevent colds and flu.

Serves: 2-3
Ingredients:
- 10 carrots sliced
- 1/2 yellow onion, diced
- 4 tablespoons minced ginger
- 2 cups vegetable broth
- 2 tablespoon
- Olive oil
- Himalayan salt to taste

Instructions:
1. First sauté onion and ginger with olive oil. Use medium heat and a large pan. Carry on until onions get translucent.
2. Then, add carrots. Stir well with sautéed onion and ginger.
3. After a couple of minutes, add the veggie broth.
4. Simmer on medium heat for about 15 minutes. Stop when the carrots get soft.
5. Finally, cool the mixture down and place through a blender. Put ingredients through blender.
6. Enjoy! This recipe is great with homemade bread that you can check out in the bonus section of the book.

Light Vegan Paleo Cucumber Salad

This salad is light, refreshing and easy to make. It's both vegan, paleo-friendly and super alkalizing, It leaves lots of room for personalization. For example, if you are super hungry, you could add some extra ingredients like red lentils and quinoa if you want to keep it vegan. You could add a hard-boiled egg if you are a vegetarian, or even some salmon or chicken to create a paleo-alkaline recipe. The choice is yours!

Serves: 2
Ingredients:
- 3 cucumbers, peeled and spiralized or thinly sliced
- 1 red onion, thinly sliced
- Juice of 1 lime
- ¼ cup coconut yoghurt or thick coconut milk/cream
- Himalayan salt and pepper to taste
- 2 tablespoons raisins
- 2 tablespoons chia seeds
- 1 tablespoon chopped cilantro
- 2 tablespoons olive oil
- 1 big avocado, peeled, pitted, sliced
- ½ cup soy sprouts or alfalfa sprouts

Instructions:
1. Combine all the ingredients in a big salad bowl (That's really it!)
2. Add protein of your choice, if desired, and enjoy.

Indian-style Potato Cakes

The Indian subcontinent is known for its inventive use of herbs and spices in countless combinations. Yum! When following a vegan, alkaline diet, it can be difficult to find sour foods. If you find yourself missing that sour, tangy taste, try this dish which uses tamarind sauce.

Servings: 4
Ingredients
- 2 cups sweet potatoes, peeled and chopped
- 1 clove of garlic, crushed
- 1 fresh red chili, finely chopped
- Salt and black pepper to taste
- 1/2 tsp ground nutmeg
- 2 tbsp fresh cilantro, chopped
- 1 tbsp lemon juice
- 3 tbsp garbanzo (chickpea) flour
- coconut oil
- Fresh cilantro to garnish

For the sauce:

- Half cup tamarind
- 1 cup boiling water
- 1 tsp fresh ginger, grated
- 1 tsp ground cumin
- 1/2 tbsp stevia

Serve with:
- 1 cup baby spinach leaves
- 1 cup chickpeas, cooked, drained and rinsed

Instructions:
1. Boil the potatoes in salted water until tender. Drain them and cool.
2. Make the tamarind sauce by pouring the boiling water over the tamarind. Simmer for 10-15 minutes and strain into a bowl.

3. Return the tamarind water to the pan and add the stevia, ginger and cumin. Bring to the boil and simmer for around 10 minutes, until thickened. Set aside until ready to use.
4. Add the potatoes, garlic, chili, salt, black pepper, nutmeg, cilantro, lemon juice and chickpea flour to a bowl. Mix them thoroughly and form the mixture into balls around the size of golf balls.
5. Flatten the balls into thick cakes and fry them on both sides in coconut oil over a low heat. This may take up to 15 minutes on each side.
6. Serve the potato cakes alongside the baby spinach leaves and chickpeas. Garnish with cilantro and drizzle the tamarind sauce over the top to finish.
7. Enjoy!

Pumpkin and Avocado Salad

Pumpkins and avocados are some of the most nutritious foods around, so what better way to enjoy them than to combine them together in this delicious salad. Avocados will provide you with a useful source of plant fats and they are also great for your skin as they are full of vitamin E.

Servings: 4
Ingredients:

- 2 cups pumpkin, peeled, deseeded and chopped
- 1 tbsp. olive oil
- 2 ripe avocados
- Lemon juice
- ½ cup baby salad leaves (your choice)

For the dressing:

- 1/2 cup vegan-friendly yogurt (e.g. coconut yoghurt or coconut cream, raw)
- 3 tbsp. fresh mint, chopped
- Half tbsp. stevia
- 1/3 tbsp. ground cumin
- Salt and black pepper to taste

Instructions

1. Preheat the oven to 400°F. (200 °C)
2. Put the pumpkin on a baking sheet and evenly coat each piece in olive oil.
3. Bake the pumpkin in the oven for 15 minutes, until soft.
4. Remove from the baking tray immediately, and set aside to cool.
5. Make the dressing by mixing all the dressing ingredients listed.
6. Peel and slice the avocado just before assembling the dish to preserve its freshness. Dress it in lemon juice to prevent it from going brown.
7. Arrange the salad starting with the leaves and then the pumpkin and avocado. Pour the dressing over the top and serve.

Spicy Zucchini Pasta with Chickpeas

This is one of my favorite recipes when I am pressed for time and hungry. A hungry woman is an angry woman! What I like about this recipe is that in the winter you can make it spicier so that it helps you warm up, whereas in the summer, you can serve it chilled, as a salad.

Servings: 2
Ingredients:
- 2 zucchini, spiralized or sliced really thin
- ½ cup chickpeas, cooked
- 1 teaspoon curry powder
- 1 teaspoon cilantro powder
- 1 onion
- Himalayan salt and black pepper to taste
- Coconut oil
- A few tablespoons of coconut milk
- Cilantro leaves to garnish
- Avocado, peeled, pitted and cut in halves
- Lemon

Instructions:
1. Heat up some coconut oil in a pan (low heat).
2. Add onion and fry gently on medium heat until translucent.
3. Add zucchini and keep stirring. Reduce the heat to low as we want to preserve all the nutrients.
4. Add chickpeas and stir well.
5. Add a bit of coconut milk as well as spices. Keep stirring.
6. Season with Himalayan salt and black pepper.
7. Turn off the heat when zucchini gets soft.
8. Serve with fresh cilantro leaves and avocado halves.
9. Sprinkle over some lemon juice.
10. Enjoy!

Super Alkaline Quinoa Gazpacho

I love this recipe when I really feel I need to alkalize in order to get more energy. This raw recipe is fantastic for the summer, however you could also heat it up if you're craving something warm. It's up to you. Quinoa is a gluten-free healthy grain and one of my favourite super foods. I always cook it in batches to make sure I have something to fall back on. Quinoa is great in all kinds of dishes- soups, stews, curries, stir-fries, smoothies and even desserts.

Servings: 2
Ingredients:
- 4 big cucumbers, peeled
- 6 big tomatoes
- ½ cup quinoa, cooked (I like to stir fry it in coconut oil and add garlic to flavour it)
- 2 tablespoons olive oil
- Himalayan salt and black pepper
- 2 garlic cloves
- Oregano and black pepper to taste

Instructions:
1. Place tomatoes, garlic and cucumbers through a juicer (I use Omega Juicer). You could also use a blender if you like it dense and with more fiber, but from my experience- if you want to add in some quinoa later on, it comes much better if you juice the ingredients instead of blending them. However both options are fine.
2. Stir well and add olive oil, quinoa, Himalayan salt, oregano and black pepper.
3. Stir again and serve.
4. Enjoy the raw energy of this dish!

For more information on quinoa (and amazing recipes), check out my article:
www.holisticwellnessproject.com/blog/health-wellness/health-benefits-of-quinoa/

Pistou Alkaline Soup

Soups and stews are the mainstay in the diets of millions of people around the world from all kinds of backgrounds. They are a nutritious and easy way to maximize the nutritional value of every single ingredient involved, as nothing is thrown away and nothing is wasted. You can enjoy these recipes at any time of day, but most of them are particularly enjoyable as those cold, winter nights close in.

What better way to spice up a simple vegetable soup than to add that French cousin of pesto that is pistou. This is a staple soup in the south of France, and absolutely packed with all kinds of vitamins, minerals and antioxidants.

Servings: 4-6
Ingredients

- 4 tbsp. olive oil
- 1 leek, finely sliced
- 4 celery stalks, diced
- 1 onion, sliced
- 3 cups seasonal, fresh vegetables, diced (for example, green beans, zucchini, artichokes, or carrots)
- 1.5 cups of cannellini beans, drained and rinsed
- handful of Bouquet garnish (mix of thyme, rosemary, bay leaves and orange peel)
- 4 cups water
- Himalayan salt and black pepper to taste

For the pistou:

- 2 cloves of garlic, chopped
- 1 tomato, chopped
- A large handful of basil leaves
- 8 tbsp. olive oil
- Himalayan Salt

Instructions:

1. Add the olive oil to a saucepan and sauté the leek, celery, onion and garlic over a medium heat.

2. Stir the mixture frequently and cook for 10 minutes, until tender.
3. Add the salt and black pepper along with the other vegetables, cannellini beans and the bouquet garni. Cook for 5 minutes.
4. Add the water and bring to the boil. Leave to simmer for 30 minutes.
5. Make the pistou by pounding the garlic and salt in a mortar. When smooth, add the tomato, basil leaves and olive oil. Make a smooth paste and set aside.
6. Serve the soup in large bowls and garnish with a big spoonful of pistou.
7. Enjoy!

Blackberry Alkaline Detox Cream

While it might sound a little unusual to make a cold soup using fruit, this dish from Georgia, Central Asia, says otherwise. It is a clever little way of using up a huge quantity of blackberries and getting a massive boost of vitamin C all at the same time. Check it out if you are not too scared to experiment with new dishes...

Servings: 4-6
Ingredients
- 3 cups fresh blackberries
- 1 clove of garlic
- Salt
- 4 tbsp. fresh cilantro, chopped
- 2 tbsp. fresh mint, chopped
- 1 cucumber, peeled and diced
- Alkaline water (optional)

Instructions:
1. First, rinse the blackberries to remove any dirt. Blend them to form a purée.
2. Force the purée through a strainer so that you end up with about 3 cups of the smoothest blackberry purée.
3. Add the garlic and a pinch of salt to a mortar and pound them until smooth.
4. Combine the garlic paste in a large bowl with the blackberry purée, cilantro, mint and half of the cucumber.
5. Refrigerate the rest of the cucumber until you want to serve the soup, which should be chilled for at least 1 hour.
6. Serve the soup cold and garnish with the rest of the cucumber pieces. Use water to experiment with a desired consistency, from a thick cream to a liquid soup, it's up to you.

Alkaline Power Soup

This soup is packed with fresh herbs like parsley, which contains massive amounts of micronutrients for such a humble leaf. It is particularly rich in iron and as such this delicious soup can be a great addition to any vegan diet. And of course- it's super alkalizing and detoxifying. Eat to your heart's content.

Servings: 4
Ingredients
- 2 tbsp. olive oil
- 2 onions, chopped
- 2 cloves of garlic, chopped
- 1 tsp fresh ginger, grated
- 1 tbsp. paprika
- 1 tsp cumin seeds
- 5 large tomatoes
- 2 cups boiling water
- Half cup of chickpeas, cooked
- 3 tbsp. fresh parsley, chopped
- 3 tbsp. celery leaves, chopped
- 3 tbsp. fresh cilantro, chopped
- 1 tbsp. lemon juice
- 1 tbsp. tomato purée
- 2 tbsp. garbanzo/ chickpea flour, slackened with 3 tbsp. water
- Salt and black pepper to taste

Instructions
1. Add the olive oil and onions to a lidded saucepan and sauté until translucent.
2. Add the garlic, ginger, paprika and cumin, sautéing them until golden.
3. Add the tomatoes and boiling water. Cover and simmer for 10 minutes, until the tomato skins begin to slough off. Remove them, taking care not to burn or scald yourself.

4. Purée the mixture with a blender and add salt and black pepper to taste.
5. Add the chickpeas, parsley, cilantro, celery leaves, lemon juice and tomato purée to the mixture.
6. Bring to the boil and allow to simmer for 5 minutes or so.
7. Use the flour mixture to thicken the mixture and then simmer for 5 more minutes.
8. Serve immediately while still hot.

Pumpkin Seed, Spinach and Tomato Soup

Pumpkin seeds are absolutely packed with zinc, magnesium and other such vital minerals essential for energy production. It's not often that we get to eat pumpkin seeds outside of a granola bar or something similar, so this recipe is definitely a keeper.

Servings: 3-4
Ingredients

- 1 cup pumpkin seeds, hulled
- 4 tbsp. water
- 4 tbsp. sunflower oil
- 1 onion, chopped
- 1 tomato, chopped
- 1/2 cup tomato purée
- 4 cups spinach (if frozen, be sure to drain and squeeze)
- 1 tsp salt
- 1/2 tsp. cayenne pepper (optional)
- 1 cup water
- Basmati rice, cooked to serve on the side

Instructions:

1. Dry fry the pumpkin seeds in a large pan over a medium heat. Keep shaking the pan and fry until golden brown. Remove from the heat and allow to cool.
2. Place the seeds in a blender with 4 tbsps. water, and blend to a paste.
3. Add the sunflower oil to a large saucepan and sauté the onion over a medium heat until golden brown.
4. Add the tomato, spinach, salt, cayenne pepper, tomato purée and 1 cup of water. Bring to the boil and reduce to a simmer.
5. Cover the saucepan and allow the mixture to cook for approximately 30 minutes. Be sure to stir it frequently.
6. Serve this thick and delicious stew with plain rice on the side.

Lentil and Basil Stew

This is a delicious stew inspired by Ethiopian cuisine, a much undervalued cuisine in the West. The generous amounts of herbs and spices included will make sure that you get a wide range of micronutrients in your diet. What's more, the lentils are an excellent source of plant protein.

Servings: 4
Ingredients

- 1 red onion, finely chopped
- 2 tbsps. olive oil
- 1 1/2 inch chunk of ginger, grated
- 2 cloves of garlic, finely chopped
- 1/2 tsp dried turmeric powder
- 1 tbsps. dried basil
- 1 cup brown lentils
- 2.5-3 cups boiling water
- 1 tsp salt
- Fresh basil to garnish, torn by hand

Instructions

1. Stir fry the onion without oil using a lidded saucepan over a medium heat. Cook for about 2 minutes, until it starts to become golden brown.
2. Lower the heat and add the olive oil, ginger, garlic, turmeric and basil. Keep stirring until the mixture is fragrant and the garlic golden. Be careful not to overdo it and burn the garlic.
3. Add the brown lentils and sauté for 1 minute. Then add the water, cover and bring to the boil.
4. Cook at a simmer for around 15 minutes. Add the salt, stir, and continue cooking until the lentils are tender.
5. Stir in the fresh basil and serve with a side of gluten free bread.

Side Dishes and Quick Snacks for Busy People

Everyone likes to have a wide range of different dishes on the table at any one time, and that's precisely what side dishes were invented for. You can use side dishes to have smaller portions of different nutrient-rich foods that would otherwise not be present at the particular meal in question. You'll find that the side dish recipes given below are tasty enough to constitute a whole meal in their own right!

Eggplant "Caviar"

Known as "Poor Man's Caviar," this is an absolutely delicious eggplant purée that you'll want to eat all day long! Eggplant is a great source of copper, vitamin B1 and fiber, and any dish that uses this deep purple beauty is worthy of including on any menu.

Servings: 2-4
Ingredients:
- 2 medium eggplants
- 2 tbsps. olive oil
- 1 onion, finely chopped
- 1 green bell pepper, deseeded and finely chopped
- 2 tbsps. tomato purée
- 4 tbsps. water
- 2 tbsps. lemon juice
- Salt and black pepper to taste
- Gluten-free bread or wrap of your choice

Instructions:
1. Pierce the eggplants several times with a sharp knife. Boil or steam them until soft. Allow them to cool.
2. Remove the stems and scoop the flesh out of the eggplants. Finely chop the soft flesh.
3. Add the olive oil to a large frying pan over a medium heat. Sauté the onion and green bell pepper until the onion is translucent.

4. Add the eggplant, tomato purée, water, salt and black pepper to the pan.
5. Reduce the heat and cook over the lowest possible heat. Stir frequently for 20-30 minutes, at which point the mixture will start to thicken.
6. Place the mixture in a bowl and stir in the lemon juice.
7. Allow the mixture to cool and place it in the fridge.
8. Serve chilled with a slice of gluten-free bread, wrap or chopped veggies (e.g. carrots or cucumbers).

Spicy Nut Mix

Owing to the fact that most fruits and vegetables are low in both fat and protein, it often falls upon nuts and seeds to pick up the shortfall in a vegan-style diets. As used in this wonderful mix, hazelnuts are also particularly rich in vitamin E and manganese which are great for your skin and overall health and wellbeing.

Serves: 4
Ingredients:
- 1/3 cup sesame seeds
- 1/2 cup hazelnuts, blanched
- 3 tbsp. coriander seeds
- 2 tbsp. cumin seeds
- Warm gluten-free tortilla wraps of your choice, sliced into strips or chopped veggies
- Olive oil
- 1/2 tsp. salt
- Black pepper to taste

Instructions
2. Dry fry the sesame seeds in a large pan over a medium heat, until they are golden. Remove from the heat and allow to cool in a bowl.
3. Toast the hazelnuts in the same pan until they are shining are starting to turn golden. Add to the sesame seeds and allow to cool.
4. Dry fry the coriander and cumin seeds until fragrant but be sure not to allow them to burn. Add them to the bowl of hazelnuts and sesame seeds and allow to cool.
5. Now put the mixture into a food processor and add salt and black pepper to taste. Process the mixture until it gains the consistency of a coarse, dry powder.
6. Serve with gluten-free tortillas wraps or veggies next to a bowl of olive oil. To consume, dip the bread or raw veggies, in the oil and then in the spicy nut mixture.

Garlic Mushrooms

Garlic is miraculous and a great source of all kinds of minerals and antioxidants. Combined with the protein-packed punch from a healthy serving of mushrooms, this dish is bound to give your mealtimes a boost. By the way, mushrooms are not really alkaline and should only be eaten sparingly as your 20-30%, but as we have already concluded, the alkaline diet is not only about eating 100% alkaline foods.

Serves: 4
Ingredients
- 2 tbsp. olive oil
- 2 cloves of garlic, crushed
- 1/4 tsp dried thyme
- 1/4 tsp dried parsley
- 1/4 tsp dried sage
- 2 cups mushrooms, chopped into quarters
- Chopped raw veggies of your choice (e.g. cucumbers, carrots, bell peppers)
- 2 tbsp. chives, chopped
- Salt and black pepper to taste

Instructions:
1. Sauté the garlic in olive oil until it softens and begins to brown.
2. Add the dried herbs and mushrooms and season with salt and black pepper to taste. Sauté this mixture over a low heat for around 10 minutes, until the mushrooms are soft.
3. Serve the mushrooms alongside raw veggies. Garnish with the chopped chives.
4. Enjoy!

Hummus

Hummus is a classic dip from the Middle East, which incorporates some of the tastiest ingredients in the region. Chickpeas provide you with a valuable source of carbohydrates and protein, while the tahini and olive oil give you a good source of healthy plant fats. It's simply delicious as a start or snack!

Ingredients:

- 1 cup cooked chickpeas, broth reserved
- 4 tbsp. light tahini
- Juice of 2 lemons
- 6 tbsp. olive oil
- 4 cloves of garlic, crushed
- Salt to taste

Instructions:

1. Blend the chickpeas with 1/8 cup of broth reserved from the cooking process.
2. Add the lemon juice, garlic, tahini and half of the olive oil.
3. Blend this mixture until smooth.
4. Leave to stand for around an hour before serving.
5. To serve, drizzle the remaining olive oil over each individual portion. Serve alongside some raw veggies.

Zucchini Vegan Paleo Hummus

This is a great option for those who follow a Paleo Diet or simply don't like legumes. All you need to do is to replace chickpeas with zucchini. I also like to add some cilantro. Zucchini can be raw or slightly cooked, it's up to you. You may even stir-fry it in coconut oil for more amazing flavour.

Ingredients:
- 1 cup zucchini slices
- 4 tbsps. light tahini
- Juice of 2 lemons
- 6 tbsps. olive oil
- 4 cloves of garlic, crushed
- Himalayan salt to taste

Instructions:
1. Combine zucchini, lemon juice, garlic, tahini and half of the olive oil in a blender.
2. Blend this mixture until smooth.
3. Leave to stand for around an hour before serving.
4. To serve, drizzle the remaining olive oil over each individual portion. Serve alongside some raw veggies or sprouted bread.

German-style Sweet Potato Salad

This healthy, alkaline version of traditional potato salad is packed with herbs, giving you a delicious source of minerals like iron and magnesium. The potatoes will give you a nice long-lasting energy boost, too!

Servings: 2-4
Ingredients:

- 2 cups sweet potatoes, chopped
- 1 cup baby spinach
- 1 cup cherry tomatoes
- 1 red bell pepper
- 4 tbsps. olive oil
- 4 scallions, trimmed and finely chopped
- 1 clove of garlic, crushed or minced
- 2 tbsps. fresh dill, finely chopped
- 2 tbsps. fresh parsley, chopped
- Salt and black pepper to taste

Instructions:

1. Clean and peel the potatoes. Boil them in a saucepan until just tender. The time required will vary depending on their size.
2. Meanwhile, sauté the garlic and scallions in a frying pan over a medium heat for 2-3 minutes, until slightly soft.
3. Add the dill and sauté for around 1 minute.
4. Remove from the heat and season to taste with the salt and black pepper.
5. Drain the potatoes once cooked, and pour the herb dressing over the top while they are hot.
6. Allow to cool and then add the rest of the ingredients and garnish with the parsley.
7. Best served chilled. Enjoy!

Quinoa Salad

This is another super quick-prep dish. Just remember to cook your quinoa in batches to be sure you always have some ready to grab from your fridge. This meal also makes an excellent take away lunch.

Serves: 2
Ingredients:
- 1 cup quinoa, cooked
- 1 garlic clove, minced
- 1 cucumber, chopped
- 1 cup fresh arugula leaves
- 1 red bell pepper, chopped
- 1 big avocado, peeled, pitted and diced
- 2 tablespoons chia seeds (optional)
- 2 tablespoons olive oil
- 2 tablespoons coconut milk (think)
- Himalayan salt and black pepper to taste
- Juice of 1 lime or lemon

Instructions:
1. Simply combine all the ingredients in a big salad bowl.
2. Toss well and sprinkle over some olive oil, coconut milk and lemon juice.
3. Enjoy!

Tasty Quinoa Coconut Salad

In case you find quinoa a bit dull, try this recipe. It will give you inspiration as for how you can experiment with all kinds of exotic flavours on the alkaline diet and transform different foods to enjoy more variety.

Serves: 2
Ingredients:

- 2 cups quinoa, cooked
- 3 tablespoons coconut oil
- 1 garlic clove, minced
- 1 teaspoon curry powder
- 1 teaspoon cilantro powder
- ½ teaspoon garlic powder
- 1 cup radish
- 1/2 cup arugula leaves
- 2 horse radishes, sliced super thin or spiralized
- ¼ cup raisins
- Himalayan salt to taste
- 1 lime

Instructions:

1. Heat some coconut oil in a pan (low or medium, heat).
2. Add garlic and sauté for a couple of minutes.
3. Then add quinoa, curry powder and garlic powder.
4. Keep stirring on low heat so that quinoa takes a nice exotic flavour.
5. Add a pinch of Himalayan salt to taste. You can also add some coconut milk.
6. Turn off the heat and let quinoa cool down.
7. In the meantime, combine the remaining ingredients in a salad bowl.
8. Add quinoa, toss well, and sprinkle over some lime juice.
9. Serve chilled.
10. Enjoy!

Mayo Alkaline Salad

If you fear eating salads because you fear you will not feel full for too long, try this one. It offers a perfect combination of refreshment that you typically get after eating a salad, but at the same time, it will keep your belly full. Notice that this salad is both vegan, alkaline and paleo friendly and leaves plenty of room for personalization in case you want to add other ingredients. Great all year long!

Serves: 4
Ingredients:

- 2 cups sweet potato, boiled, sliced, chilled
- 1 cup soy sprouts (I am not talking about soy, but soy sprouts...)
- 2 red bell peppers, chopped
- 1 onion, chopped
- 1 cup arugula leaves
- ¼ cup almond, crushed
- ½ cup vegan mayonnaise
- Juice of 1 lime
- 2 tablespoons olive oil
- Himalayan salt and black pepper to taste

Instructions:

1. Combine all the ingredients in a big salad bowl.
2. Add vegan mayo, olive oil, lemon juice, black pepper and salt.
3. Mix well. Cool down in a refrigerator for a couple of hours.
4. Serve chilled and enjoy!

Black-eyed Peas and Orange Salad

It's becoming increasingly popular to include fruit as part of an otherwise savoury salad. This is great for us "alkalarians" as it adds another nutritional dimension to the dish. Oranges, even though not super alkalizing, are well known for being high in vitamin C and make a great accompaniment to the protein-rich black-eyed peas. Balanced diet is the key to success. We should not fear fruit.

Servings: 4
Ingredients:
- 1 cup black-eyed peas, soaked
- 1 bay leaf
- A slice of onion
- Zest and juice of 1 orange
- 5 tbsp. olive oil
- 6 large olives, pitted and chopped
- 4 scallions, trimmed and chopped
- 2 tbsp. fresh parsley, chopped
- 2 tbsp. fresh basil, chopped
- 4 whole oranges
- 1 large handful of watercress

Instructions
1. Put the black-eyes peas, bay leaf and onion slice in a saucepan filled with enough water to cover them by 1 inch.
2. Boil at a high heat for 10 minutes, then reduce to a simmer and cook for 60 minutes, until the black-eyed peas are soft.
3. Whisk the olive oil, orange rind and juice in a bowl.
4. Add the olives, scallions and herbs, then mix.
5. Drain the black-eyed peas and add them to the mixture.
6. Season to taste and ensure that the black-eyed peas are well-coated by the mixture.
7. Serve the mixture on individual plates, and add some orange segments and a pile of watercress to each.

Quick Alka-Goulash

Inspired the Hungarian classic of the same name, this speedy version of Goulash is a flavor explosion! The generous portion of cooked tomatoes included mean that you'll be getting plenty of antioxidants, lycopene in particular.

Servings: 4
Ingredients:
- 1 onion, finely chopped
- 1 clove of garlic, crushed
- 2 carrots, diced
- 3 zucchini, diced
- 2 tbsp. olive oil
- 1 tbsp. paprika
- 1/4 tsp. ground nutmeg
- 1 tbsp. fresh parsley, chopped
- 1 tbsp. tomato purée
- 2 cups of tomatoes, peeled
- 2 cups cooked red kidney beans, drained and rinsed
- 1/2 cup tomato juice
- Salt and black pepper to taste

Instructions
1. Sauté the onion, garlic, carrot and zucchini in olive oil over a medium heat for 5 minutes, until softened.
2. Stir in the paprika, nutmeg, parsley and tomato puree.
3. Add the tomatoes, red kidney beans and tomato juice, and stir.
4. Simmer for 10 minutes until warmed through.
5. Serve immediately. Enjoy!

Pea Risotto

One of the great classics of rice-based cuisine, risotto is often made with the addition of butter or some kind of meat or poultry which are acid-forming. Fortunately, this simply doesn't have to be the case. A perfectly delicious risotto can be made without any of these things in a more alkaline friendly and vegan way.

Servings: 4
Ingredients:
- 1 vegetable broth cube
- 2 tbsp. olive oil
- 1 onion, finely chopped
- 3 cloves of garlic, finely chopped
- 1 cup basmati rice
- 1 cup frozen peas
- 1 cup fresh baby spinach leaves
- 1 lemon, grated and juiced
- Salt and black pepper to taste
- 3 cups water

Instructions
1. Crumble the vegetable broth cube into 3 cups of boiling water. Allow it to dissolve and then reduce the heat.
2. Defrost the peas in warm water, drain and set aside for later.
3. Season the onion with salt and black pepper to taste, and then sauté it in olive oil at a medium heat for around 5 minutes, until softened.
4. Add the garlic to the frying pan and sauté for a few minutes, ensuring that it doesn't burn.
5. Add the rice to the frying pan and mix well. Ladle in some vegetable broth so that the rice is just covered.
6. Simmer over medium heat while constantly stirring for a few minutes, until the liquid has been almost completely absorbed.
7. Add the rest of the broth a ladleful at a time, stirring constantly until each batch of broth has been absorbed.

8. After each ladleful has been absorbed and the rice is fully cooked, add the defrosted peas, baby spinach leaves and lemon juice.
9. Stir until the baby spinach leaves have wilted and then serve while hot.
10. Enjoy!

Satisfying Alka-Lunch Paleo Smoothie

I know what you're thinking. Is Marta putting her alkaline breakfast recipes into a lunch cookbook? Well, I can understand your confusion and usually I don't have smoothies for lunch, however I think there is nothing wrong with that. Especially if you are pressed for time. This is what I do whenever I am in rush; I just make myself a satisfying, nutritious smoothie that keeps me full till my mid-afternoon snack or sometimes even until dinner!

Servings: 1-2
Ingredients:
- 1 big avocado
- 1.5 cup coconut milk or almond milk
- 2 tablespoons fresh cilantro leaves
- 2 tablespoons coconut oil
- 1 lemon, juiced
- 4 tablespoons of chia seeds
- Himalayan salt to taste

Instructions:
1. Simply blend all the ingredients except seeds and oil.
2. Stir well, add chia seeds and taste with Himalayan salt.
3. Enjoy!

BONUS RECIPES
Tempting Afternoon Treats (gluten-free, dairy-free and virtually sugar-free)

Everyone likes a treat now and again, even the most health-minded of folk. I believe we can have both health and pleasure of treating ourselves to delicious treats. With this in mind, we have compiled some of the most delectable recipes we could think of for your perusal. Whatever your tastes, you're sure to find a dessert to suit you and your family. Following an alkaline diet doesn't have to limit your choices and you'll see how in this chapter. In case you happen to have a sweet tooth during the afternoon, you will have a list of excellent guilty free treats to satisfy it. So much better than to rely on will power alone, right?

Raspberries with Baked Apples

Fruits are amazing for providing all sorts of vitamins and minerals, all in a delicious, sweet and natural package. Even though most fruits are not considered "alkaline-forming" (because they are rich in sugar), they provide an excellent alternative to processed baked foods, cake and chocolate. This is a perfect treat to enjoy on your 30%!

Don't get too paranoid about fruit. For example, if you can choose between a processed chocolate bar and an apple, apple is a much better choice. At the same time, remember not to eat fruit in excess. Try to stick more with alkaline forming fruit (no sugar) like limes, lemons, grapefruits etc.

Servings: 6
Ingredients
- 2 tbsp. lemon juice
- 4 tbsp. water
- 1 tsp. stevia (optional)
- 1 tsp cinnamon
- 3 dessert apples
- 1 cup raspberries

Instructions:

1. Preheat the oven to 400°F. (200°C)
2. Add the lemon juice, water and stevia to a bowl and mix them well to make a sauce.
3. Halve and core each apple using your preferred method.
4. Coat each apple half in the sauce mixture. Reserve the remaining sauce.
5. Bake the apples in an ovenproof dish for around 25 minutes, until they begin to soften.
6. Remove the apples from the oven and cover them with the raspberries.
7. Pour the remainder of the apple sauce over the fruit.
8. Reduce the oven temperature to 300 degrees F (150 degrees Celsius) , then bake the fruit for 10 minutes.
9. Serve immediately, while still hot.

Baked Bananas with Pear and Orange Sauce

Bananas are a wonderful source of potassium and one of the few commonly eaten fruits which contains a reasonable source of plant fats. When ripe, bananas are delectably sweet and make a perfect dessert when combined with a pear and orange sauce as below. Like already mentioned, even though most fruit, like for example, fruit rich in sugar (like bananas) is not considered alkaline, it doesn't have to be rejected forever as it forms part of a balanced diet and is packed with nutrients. We need to remember that the alkaline diet is all about balance, it's not about eating 100% alkaline meals all the time. Just aim for 70% alkaline and leave room for other foods as well. Remember that I have downloadable, printable charts for you to make your life easier and you can download them at: www.bitly.com/AlkalineMarta

Servings: 4
Ingredients:

- 2 oranges
- 2 ripe pears
- 4 bananas
- Stevia to taste

Instructions:

1. Preheat the oven to 350 degrees F. (175 degrees Celsius)
2. Remove and slice the rind from one of the oranges into strips, taking care to avoid the white pith.
3. Blanch the orange strips in boiling water for around 3 minutes, just to soften them up. Drain them and set aside.
4. Peel this orange and remove the segments and set aside.
5. Use the other orange for its juice, squeezing it out and setting it aside for later.
6. Peel and core the pears and place them with the organs juice in a blender. Blend until smooth. Sweeten with stevia if you wish.

7. Peel the bananas and place them in an ovenproof dish. Pour the pear sauce over the top.
8. Cover and bake for 15 minutes, until the bananas are soft.
9. Decorate with the orange segments and orange peel. Serve right away, while still hot.
10. Enjoy!

Almost Alkaline Blueberry Muffins

One of the all-time classics of the dessert world, blueberry muffins are ubiquitous in cafés and dessert rooms throughout the globe. Alkalarians don't have to be excluded from the often dairy-rich environment that is dessert making. Try this delicious recipe that is vegan-friendly and even gluten-free!

Servings: 4
Ingredients:
- ½ cup almond flour
- ¼ cup almonds, ground
- ¼ cup desiccated coconut
- 1/2 tsp bicarbonate of soda
- 3/4 tsp baking powder
- 1 banana, mashed
- ½ cup almond milk
- 1 tsp vanilla extract
- 1 cup blueberries
- Muffin cases

Instructions:
1. Preheat the oven to 350°F. (175 Celsius)
2. Combine the gram flour, almonds, desiccated coconut, bicarbonate of soda and baking powder in a bowl.
3. In a separate bowl, whisk the mashed banana with the almond milk and vanilla extract.
4. Make a well in the middle of the flour mixture and slowly pour the milk mixture into it. Fold them mixture from the edges towards the middle to incorporate the milk into the batter. Be sure to be gentle at this point.
5. Add the blueberries and fold them gently into the batter.
6. Spoon the batter into muffin cases, leaving a gap of about 1/2 inch at the top.
7. Bake for around 20-25 minutes, until the muffins have risen properly and cooked through.
8. Set aside to cool slightly. Consume either warm or cold, as you prefer.

Not-So-Alkaline Chocolate Brownies

There's nothing quite like a chocolate brownie! Let's not pretend that they're particularly nutritious, but this recipe does at least contain plenty of walnuts and dark, vegan-friendly dark chocolate for a hefty amount of minerals and micronutrients. In any case, you deserve to treat yourself occasionally and that's what this chapter is all about after all.

Servings: 8
Ingredients:
- 2 cups almond flour
- 1 tsp baking powder
- Dash of Himalayan salt
- 1 banana, mashed
- 1/2 tsp. stevia (optional)
- 1 tbsp. vanilla extract
- Half cup dark raw chocolate, broken up
- 4 tbsps. vegan-friendly margarine or coconut oil
- 1 tbsps. stevia
- ¼ cup dark chocolate chips
- ½ cup walnuts, chopped

Instructions:
1. Preheat the oven to 360°F (180 Celsius). Grease an 8 inch baking tin using vegan-friendly margarine or coconut oil.
2. Use a sieve to sift the all-purpose white flour, salt and baking powder into a bowl.
3. In a separate bowl, combine the mashed banana, stevia, caster sugar and vanilla extract. Mix until smooth.
4. Bring a saucepan of water to the boil and then bring it back down to a simmer. Place a glass bowl on top of the saucepan. Melt the dark chocolate, vegan-friendly margarine in the bowl.
5. Pour the melted chocolate mixture into the banana purée. Mix well.

6. Make a well in the middle of the flour and add the chocolate mixture slowly, folding it into the flour as you go along.
7. Add the dark chocolate chips and chopped walnuts, mixing them gently into the brownie batter.
8. Pour the brownie batter into the prepared baking tin.
9. Bake for around 25 minutes, or until the brownie reach your favourite consistency.
10. Once completely cool, divide the slab of brownie into 12 equal squares.
11. Enjoy!

Alka-Paleo-Vegan Ice Cream

One of the first things that novice alkalarians will think that they'll miss out on is ice cream. Luckily for them, that's just a misconception and not at all the case. We can enjoy various kinds of vegan ice cream which are practically indistinguishable from the dairy kind. Believe it or not, but this recipe actually uses lots of healthy spices with anti-inflammatory properties and is sugar free (stevia is not sugar).

Servings: 4
Ingredients:
- 2 cups coconut milk
- ½ cup coconut cream
- 1/4 cup stevia powder
- 1/4 tsp ground cinnamon
- 1/4 tsp ground nutmeg
- 1/4 tsp ground allspice
- 1 teaspoon vanilla powder
- 1/2 cup cashew butter or almond butter

Optional (to serve)
- lemon or lime juice
- raisins
- Maca powder
- Chia seeds
- Barley grass powder or alfalfa powder to alkalize and detoxify

Instructions:
1. Blend the coconut milk, cream and cashew butter until smooth.
2. Add the stevia, cinnamon, nutmeg and allspice berries.
3. Transfer the mixture to an ice cream dish and freeze overnight or until firm.
4. Enjoy!

Alka-Paleo Vegan Coco Biscuits

I love those homemade biscuits as a healthy, gluten-free snack. This recipe is vegan, alkaline and even paleo friendly. Moreover, you can experiment with different spices and tastes. This recipe serves to help you satisfy your sweet tooth, however, you could also use curry powder and other herbs to make it spicy.

Servings: 10

Ingredients:

- 4 cups of coconut flour
- ¼ cup organic sugar or stevia
- 1 ½ tablespoons of baking powder
- Half teaspoon of Himalayan salt
- 1 ½ cups of unsweetened almond milk
- 1 cup of coconut oil (room temperature)

Instructions:

1. Preheat your oven to a temperature of 400°F (200 Celsius).
2. Using a small bowl, combine the flour with stevia, baking powder and Himalayan salt.
3. Stir the ingredients well and add in raw almond milk. Whisk energetically so that the mixture is smooth.
4. Using your hands, start shaping the mixture into small biscuits.
5. Place them on a parchment-lined baking sheet and bake them for 16 to 20 minutes so that they are slightly golden in color.
6. Cool them down, serve and enjoy!

Alkaline Cinnamon Pumpkin Bread

This one is one of my favorite pumpkin recipes and one of my favorite healthy comfort foods!

Servings: around 8
Ingredients:

- 1 ½ tablespoons of ground flaxseed
- 2 ½ tablespoons of warm alkaline water
- 1 ½ cups of pumpkin puree
- 1/4 cup of organic cane sugar (or stevia)
- 3 tablespoons of melted coconut oil
- 1 tablespoon of baking powder
- 1 ½ teaspoons of ground cinnamon
- ½ teaspoon of ground nutmeg
- Pinch of Himalayan salt
- ¾ cups of raw, unsweetened almond milk
- 1 ½ cups of almond flour
- 1 cup of coconut flour
- 1 ¼ cups of gluten-free oats

Instructions:

1. Preheat your oven to 350°F.
2. Place some parchment on the bottom of a loaf pan.
3. Spray the rest of a pan with cooking spray.
4. In a bowl, combine water with flaxseed.
5. Let it sit for about 5 minutes.
6. In the meantime, in another bowl, combine the pumpkin puree, stevia or sugar, coconut oil, baking powder, cinnamon, nutmeg, and Himalayan salt.
7. Now add in the flaxseed mixture from step 4. Add almond milk until well combined.
8. Using another utensil, stir the almond flour together with coconut flour and oats.
9. Finally, combine the dry ingredients with the wet ingredient mix stirring it into a batter.
10. Pour the batter into your loaf pan.
11. Bake the pumpkin bread around 1 hour, until a knife that you insert in the middle comes out clean.

12. Cool down for half an hour, serve and enjoy with a nice cup of herbal chai tea!

Alkaline Vegan Milk Recipes (Home-Made)

Of all vegan milk we can create, almond milk is certainly my favorite. Personally, I am not a big fan of soy milk, because large amounts don't agree with my stomach (even though I have always stuck to organic options). I have also experimented with rice milk, but I finally discovered an even more natural, nutritious, and raw (aside from coconut milk that I always praise) is raw almond milk. You can make your own and save money. Besides, if you make your own, you always know its ingredients. I remember looking for almond milk in bio supermarkets and in organic stores where I live. To my disappointment, most of them had added sugar (even though they had an "organic" label on them), and those that didn't were extremely expensive. This predicament has driven me to create my own rituals and make my own almond milk. Try it yourself! Almond milk is also Paleo-friendly (for those of you who follow Paleo) while soy milk and rice milk aren't. Still, when I was starting on my dairy-free journey, I would try different options to see what worked for me. Lesson learned-almond milk rocks!

After you have created this recipe, store your milk in a fridge. Almond milk will keep up to one week.

Almond Milk Recipe
Serves: 4 cups
Ingredients:
- 4 cups filtered, preferably alkaline water
- 1 cup of raw almonds
- ½ teaspoon Himalayan salt or sea salt
- A few dates or 2 tablespoons of maple syrup

Instructions:
1. First, soak almonds in water with ½ salt (sea salt or Himalayan salt) for about 12 hours.
2. Place in a high speed blender until the mixture is smooth.

3. Strain using cheesecloth.
4. Place in a blender again, adding some pitted dates or maple syrup.
5. Stir well and place in a fridge.
6. Serve with a splash of lemon or lime juice or some fresh cinnamon. So yummy, healthy and nutritious!

Coconut Milk Recipe

I realize that some people may be allergic to nuts, or for whatever reason, don't like them. I want to invite you to try some homemade raw coconut milk instead. Just like almond milk, you can use it in cooking, baking, smoothies, and other natural drinks. You can experiment with cocoa, vanilla, dried fruits, and strawberries to give it some flavor.

Serves: 4
Ingredients:
- 4 cups of warm water
- 2 cups shredded coconut

Instructions:
1. I recommend you make this recipe in 2 batches.
2. First, take 1 cup of coconut and 2 cups of water and place in a blender. Keep blending for a few minutes until smooth.
3. Strain using a colander and set aside. Keep the strained coconut as well. You can use it for desserts or add it back to your milk.
4. Now, blend the second batch. Place another 2 cups of water and 1 cup of shredded coconut in the blender.
5. Blend well.
6. Mix the two batches and, if needed, add some of the blended coconut for more thickness.
7. Sweeten with stevia, maple syrup or blend again with some dried fruit.
8. Enjoy!

BONUS II Transition Recipes. Paleo and Vegetarian Alkaline Lunch Recipes

Tuna Salad

Servings: 2-3
Ingredients:
- 1 can of paleo albacore tuna, drained
- 2 tablespoons of cashew nuts
- 1/4 cup of chopped tomatoes
- 2 cups of baby spinach
- 2-3 tablespoons of homemade paleo pesto (simply blend some olive oil with Himalaya salt and fresh basil leaves and tomato juice)
- 1/4 cup of chopped bell peppers

Instructions:
1. Take drained tuna in a bowl. Add the bell peppers, spinach, cashew nuts and tomatoes to the tuna.
2. Toss the drained tuna mixture with pesto. Serve.
3. Enjoy!

Vegetarian Salad with an Alkaline Twist

Servings: 2-3
Ingredients:

- 1 can of tuna, drained
- 2 tablespoons of cashew nuts
- 1/4 cup of chopped tomatoes
- 2 cups of baby spinach
- 2-3 tablespoons of homemade paleo pesto (simply blend some olive oil with Himalaya salt and fresh basil leaves and tomato juice)
- 1/4 cup of chopped bell peppers

Method of preparation:
1. Take drained tuna in a bowl. Add the bell peppers, spinach, cashew nuts and tomatoes to the tuna.
2. Toss the drained tuna mixture with pesto. Serve.
3. Enjoy!

Spanish Aioli

Make sure you use this dip with fish and seafood...absolutely delicious! Garlic is just miraculous and it is a natural antibiotic. Eating raw garlic is not always practical, however you can add it as a wonderful, tasty dip!

Ingredients:
- 7 cloves of garlic, chop
- 1/2 tsp. salt
- 1 tsp. freshly squeezed lemon juice
- 2 eggs (yolks only)
- 2/3 cup olive oil
- 1 tablespoon fresh oregano, chop

Instructions:
1. Put your oregano, salt and the garlic into the processor and mix well.
2. Put in the lemon juice and egg, pulse again.
3. Slowly drizzle the oil into the food processor and pulse well.

You can serve with fish, bread, zucchini, fries or the kale chips below.

Spicy Salmon with Chopped Almonds and Lemon

Serves: 2
Ingredients:
- 2 slices of cooked salmon
- Bite-sized lettuce (3 cups)
- Spinach leaves, chopped (2 cups)
- Minced red onions (1 cup)
- Lemon juice (2 tbsps.)
- Olive Oil (2 tbsps.)
- Chopped almonds (1 cup)
- Himalayan salt, to taste
- Black Pepper, to taste
- Chili powder, to taste
- Coconut milk or cream (about 2 tbsps.)
- A few cherry tomatoes and radishes for garnish

Instructions:
1. Combine salmon, bite-sized lettuce, spinach, and minced red onions in a bowl.
2. Pour lemon juice and olive oil into the bowl. Add some black pepper, chili powder, Himalayan salt and coconut milk.
3. Add chopped almonds.
4. Season with Himalaya salt and chili powder.
5. Garnish with tomatoes and radishes. Add a couple of lime slices and serve.
6. Enjoy!

Tomato Garlic Soup

Serves: 2
Ingredients:
- 2 hard-boiled eggs, mashed
- 4 garlic cloves, peeled
- 8 big tomatoes, peeled
- Filtered water (preferably alkaline)
- Himalaya Salt
- Coconut milk
- Black pepper
- Ginger powder
- 1 tablespoon parsley
- 1 tablespoon cilantro
- Optional: green, alkaline powders

Instructions:
1. Blend tomatoes and garlic.
2. Heat up the mixture in a pot, (low heat) and add 2 tablespoons of olive oil and some water.
3. Stir well and add 2 pinches of Himalaya salt, black pepper, ginger, cilantro and parsley. Add more water if necessary.
4. Finally, add the eggs and stir well. If you like it creamy, add a few tablespoons of coconut milk.
5. Serve slightly warm. I also have it chilled and raw in the summer! Add some alkaline powders (for example alfalfa) to make it even more nutritious and alkaline
6. Enjoy!

Afterword- Stay Alkaline

The aim of this recipe book was to show you how you can adapt to a clean alkaline diet. This alkaline inspired cuisine allows you to still eat mouth-watering, healthy, wholesome meals that will enable you to live life to the fullest without feeling deprived.

You will find the recipes to suit all kinds of occasions and all sorts of palates. If you have already tried out a recipe or two on a friend or family member who are new to alkaline way of eating, I bet you were not particularly surprised when they asked for an exact recipe!

Hopefully, you'll continue to get a lot of use out of this book as you progress with your alkaline diet lifestyle returning again and again to your favourite recipes. Here's wishing you all the best in your health and wellness journey!

Book 3
The Alkaline Diet Lifestyle Cookbook Vol.3

Irresistible Alkaline Dinner Recipes for Natural Weight Loss, Healing, and Supercharged Health

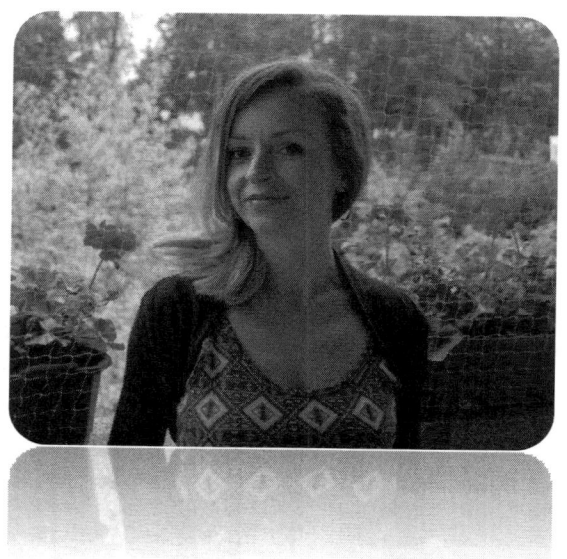

www.HolisticWellnessProject.com
www.amazon.com/author/mtuchowska

Amazing Alkaline-Friendly Dinners

Eating alkaline is easier than you can imagine, especially if you have a set of delicious and easy-to-make recipes. Evening is a time of the day when we are very prone to all kinds of unhealthy temptations, simply because we feel a bit tired and very often stressed. Luckily, the alkaline diet can take care of you with a whole variety of tasty and nutritious dinner recipes. You can pick and choose between vegan, vegetarian and even Paleo (still 70-80% alkaline) options depending on your mood. With this recipe book, you will be looking forward to celebrating dinner time with your family, friends and, of course, your favorite healthy foods. My number 1 suggestion is: always try to have some healthy, guilt-free snacks for late afternoon and early evening. It can be a real lifesaver and can actually make you reconsider the desire to order some pizza or take away food. Since most people are busy or tired in the evenings, it's better (and safer) to make sure that you cook in batches (for example on weekends), plan your meals and always have some veggies that are ready to grab (washed and chopped). This is a fantastic plan to minimize the time you spend in the kitchen or shopping. Planning is the key. Recommended Resources (article + recipes + audio) www.holisticwellnessproject.com/blog/alkaline-diet/alkaline-lifestyle-for-busy-people/

Many of my readers and clients told me that evening time was the most difficult time to "stay healthy" as they all had uncontrollable food cravings and just felt like giving in to eating bad. This is something I can definitely relate to as I had this problem in the past and it would spoil all my alkaline diet efforts. The solution is quite simple:

1. Stop "going hungry". You see, many people focus on eliminating certain foods first instead of adding. The way I see it is like this: focus on adding more alkaline foods first and then start gradually eliminating acidic foods that do not support your health goals.
2. Do not skip breakfast and always eat lunch.
3. Be sure to carry some alkaline snacks, like nuts and seeds, with you.

4. Try to have a small mid-afternoon meal. Here in Spain, where I currently live, they call it "merienda," in Poland, where I am originally from, they call it "podwieczorek" (such a difficult word, I know!). I usually grab a smoothie, a simple veggie wrap or some homemade gluten-free bakes. I usually have 5 meals a day (yes!), breakfast, mid-morning snack, lunch, mid-afternoon snack and dinner. Golden rule - it's not about eating less; it's about eating right. If you follow this rule, you will make it to evening time feeling nicely energized and really motivated to carry on a healthy track. Heck, with this 5 meals a day routine, I can even have a nice evening walk before or after my dinner. The energy you get from eating more alkaline is amazing, and I am absolutely passionate about helping you experience it in a doable, easy, fun and practical way!

Once you've learned some of the recipes in this section, dinner will never be a bore again. In many parts of the world, animal products are hard to come by and people have had to rely on naturally vegan foods by necessity rather than choice. We can make the most of these recipes and their invariably nutritious content by using them to make tasty evening meals for everyone in the family.

Alkaline Dinners
SECTION I Alkaline Vegan Recipes
Vegetable Paella

Unlike most forms of paella, this dish is completely vegan-friendly. It contains everything you could ask for from a single dish and can be eaten with great pleasure at any time of year.

Serves: 4-6
Ingredients:
- 3 tbsp. olive oil
- 1 onion, finely chopped
- 1 eggplant, finely chopped
- 1 zucchini, finely chopped
- 1 red bell pepper, finely chopped
- 3 cloves of garlic, finely chopped
- 2 tomatoes, chopped
- 1 tsp smoked paprika
- 1 1/3 cups paella (Arborio) rice
- 6 cups boiling water
- Pinch of saffron
- 2/3 cup green beans, finely chopped
- 2/3 cup peas

Instructions:
1. Add the olive oil to a large frying pan and sauté the onion, eggplant, zucchini and red bell pepper over a medium heat until golden.
2. Add the garlic and cook for 1 minute, until fragrant.
3. Add the tomatoes, rice and smoked paprika.
4. Stir and then add half the water along with the saffron and some salt and black pepper to taste.
5. Stir the mixture and then cover and increase the heat.
6. Cook at a high heat for 10 minutes, ensuring that you don't burn anything.
7. Add the remainder of the water, stir and cover. Reduce the heat to medium and cook for 20 minutes. Do not stir at this point.

167

8. Add the green beans and peas for the final 5 minutes of cooking.
9. The rice ought to be *al dente* (=firm) when ready. Leave to stand for 5 minutes and then serve while still hot.
10. Enjoy!

Tofu in Black Bean Sauce

While many of you may choose not to consume soya products, it can be an important protein source for those who do enjoy the occasional piece of tofu. As such, this recipe has been included in this book with the intention of inclusivity in mind. The wide variety of mushrooms used in such dishes (even though not alkaline) can be a great source of vitamin D.

Serves: 4
Ingredients:
- 1 cup dried mushrooms (shiitake mushrooms are particularly delicious)
- 3/4 cup boiling water
- 1 cup fresh firm tofu
- 3 tbsps. coconut oil
- 4 green bell peppers, chopped
- 1 large fresh chili pepper, deseeded and sliced
- 2 cloves of garlic, sliced
- 1 tbsp. cornstarch

+Boiled brown rice or quinoa to serve on the side

For the sauce:
- 2 tsp black bean sauce
- 3 tbsps. Bragg Liquid Aminos
- 1 tbsp. hoisin sauce
- 1 tbsp. tomato purée

Instructions:
1. Place the mushrooms in a bowl and add the boiling water. Leave them for 30 minutes to become reconstituted.
2. Reserve the water from the mushrooms. Slice the mushrooms and add the sauce ingredients.
3. Drain the tofu and wrap in paper towels to absorb any excess liquid. When you are ready, cut them into 3/4 inch pieces.

4. Add the sunflower oil to a wok placed over a high heat. Add the mushrooms, green bell pepper, chili and garlic and stir fry for 2 minutes. Be sure not to burn the garlic.
5. Add the sauce mixture and stir the contents of the wok continuously for about 2 minutes, until the sauce is thickened.
6. Add the cornstarch to the cool mushroom water, stir, and then pour into the wok.
7. Stir the mixture over the wok until thick, and then add the tofu, stirring until it has been coated with the sauce and warmed through.
8. Serve immediately with a side of boiled rice.

One Pot Beans

Beans are one of the most important sources of protein for those of us following a vegan way of life, and this dish makes them simply delicious. This recipe is great for when those cold, winter nights are drawing in.

Serves: 4
Ingredients:
- 2 tbsps. olive oil
- 2 vegetable stock cubes, crumbled
- 2 onions, chopped
- 2 apples, peeled and grated
- 2 carrots, grated
- 3 tbsps. tomato purée
- 1 cup water
- 1 tsp dried oregano
- 1 tsp ground cumin
- 2 cups red kidney beans, pre-cooked
- Salt and black pepper to taste

Instructions:
1. Preheat the oven to 350°F. (175 Celsius)
2. Sauté the onion, stock cubes, apple and carrot in a frying pan over a medium heat for 5 minutes, stirring constantly.
3. Mix the tomato purée into the water. Add this, the dried oregano, and ground cumin to the sautéed mixture and stir well.
4. Cover and simmer for about 2 minutes.
5. Add the red kidney beans, stir, and pour the whole mixture into a casserole dish.
6. Cover and cook in the oven for about 40 minutes. Add a little extra water if the mixture starts to look dry.
7. Serve while still hot.

Sweet Potato Cottage Pie

Cottage pie is one of those homely classics, perfect at any time of year as a bit of comfort food. This version consists of an all vegan filling and uses sweet potato as the topping, rather than the more conventional white potato. This way, you get a source of starchy goodness with a healthy dose of vitamin A to top it off. That's not something the average white potato could do!

Serves: 6
Ingredients:
For the filling:

- 1 tbsp. olive oil
- 1 leek, finely chopped
- 1 parsnip, diced
- 1 carrot, diced
- 1 celery stalk, diced
- 2 cloves of garlic, minced
- 2 cups canned tomatoes
- 1 tbsp. tomato purée
- 2 cups green lentils, cooked, drained and rinsed
- 1 cup frozen peas
- Salt and black pepper

For the topping:

- 4 medium sweet potatoes, chopped
- 1 tsp vegan margarine or coconut oil
- ¼ cup fresh dill, chopped

Instructions:

1. Sauté the onion, leek, carrot and parsnip in olive oil until the vegetables begin to soften.
2. Add the garlic to the frying pan and season with salt and black pepper to taste.
3. Add the tomatoes, tomato purée and simmer for 20 minutes. Add some water if the consistency is too thick.
4. To make the sweet potato mash, boil the sweet potato in salted water for 20 minutes, until it is soft. Drain and mash with the vegan margarine.

5. Stir the dill into the mashed sweet potato and return to the heat, cooking gently for around 5 minutes, until the mixture begins to firm up. Set aside when ready.
6. Preheat the oven to 360°F. (180 Celsius).
7. Add the drained and rinsed green lentils to the tomato sauce. Add the frozen peas and cook for 5 minutes until fully heated through.
8. Transfer the filling to an 8 inch baking dish. Top the filling with the sweet potato mixture, ensuring that it is covered completely.
9. Bake for around 30 minutes, until the cottage pie is bubbling in the oven.
10. Leave the dish to cool for around 10 minutes, then serve and enjoy.

Sweet Potato Wedges with a Twist

Very easy dish that helps you sneak in some green, alkalizing and hydrating veggies in the form of spiralized zucchinis.

Servings: 4 to 6
Ingredients:
- 6 large sweet potatoes, peeled and cut in wedges
- 4 tablespoons coconut oil
- 1 teaspoon smoked paprika + other spices of your choice (curry also works great!)
- Himalayan salt to taste
- 2 zucchinis, sliced very thinly with a spiralizer

Instructions:
1. Preheat the oven to a temperature of 450°F (230 Celsius) and line two rimmed baking sheets with parchment.
2. Mix the sweet potatoes with some coconut oil adding the spices and Himalayan salt.
3. Place the potatoes in a single layer on top of the rimmed baking sheets.
4. Start baking and keep stirring occasionally. When almost done (after about 15 minutes) add the spiraled or sliced zucchinis and keep baking for 5 minutes more until soft.
5. Cool for 5 minutes and serve with some greens on side.

Easy Vegan Burger

This is my favorite vegan-alkaline fast food!

Servings: 4
Ingredients:
- 2 large red bell peppers, chopped
- Coconut oil
- Salt and pepper to taste
- 4 vegan sandwich buns, preferable gluten-free or sprouted, toasted
- 4 tablespoons fresh basil pesto
- 1 cup fresh arugula

Instructions:
1. Stir fry the red bell peppers in coconut oil adding Himalayan salt and spices of your choice.
2. Set aside when ready.
3. Spread some pesto on the top half of each sandwich bun.
4. Place the stir-fried red bell peppers onto the bottom half of each sandwich bun.
5. Top with fresh arugula and the top half of the buns.
6. Serve warm.
7. Enjoy!

Easy Red Pepper Hummus

This hummus can be a real life-saver. If you are too busy to cook or too tired after work, you can just satisfy your hunger in a healthy way. Hummus is great to serve with raw veggies as well as in all kinds of wraps.

Servings: 10 to 12

Ingredients:
- 1 cup chickpeas, cooked, rinsed and drained
- 1/4 cup of roasted red peppers, chopped
- 3 cloves minced garlic
- ½ jalapeno, seeded and minced
- Himalayan Salt and pepper to taste
- 4 tablespoons olive oil
- Water, as needed
- 2 tbsps. fresh cilantro
- Juice of 1 lime

Instructions:
7. Combine the chickpeas, cilantro, roasted red pepper, garlic and jalapeno in a food processor and blend until super smooth.
8. Add in some olive oil, lime juice, and water to achieve the desired consistency and blend again.
9. Add Himalayan salt and pepper to taste, mix well and serve as a dip with some raw veggies or sprouted bread/wraps. Enjoy!

Alkaline Comfort Tomato Soup

Tomatoes are miraculous and highly alkalizing. They are one of my favorite alkaline common-sense super foods!

Serves: 2-4
Ingredients:

- 3 cups of fresh tomatoes, peeled (immerse in some warm water to get the peel off)
- 4 leeks thinly sliced
- 6 garlic cloves, minced
- 2 tablespoons coconut oil
- 1 cup vegetable broth
- 1 can coconut milk or almond milk
- Salt and fresh pepper or other spices to taste

Instructions:

1. Using a large saucepan, sauté leeks in some oil (medium heat) until translucent.
2. Add garlic and stir together for 1 minute. Switch off the heat.
3. In the meantime, blend the peeled tomatoes in a blender.
4. Add the mixture to your saucepan and put on low heat. Stir well.
5. Add coconut milk, vegetable broth, salt and spices.
6. Simmer on low heat until warm and serve.
7. Enjoy!

Easy Tomato Salad

The easiest way to get more alkaline is to simply add more raw foods into your diet, especially alkaline fruits and vegetables. It's not that you have to survive on salads alone, but if you just choose to serve some salads with your main meals, you will certainly see a difference.

Serves: 4
Ingredients:

- 1 small shallot, thinly sliced
- 4-5 medium tomatoes, sliced
- 2 cucumbers, peeled and spiralizer
- ½ cup alfalfa sprouts
- 6 medium basil leaves
- Himalayan salt
- Freshly ground pepper
- Juice of 1 lime
- Olive oil or avocado oil

Instructions:

1. Combine all the ingredients in a salad bowl, toss well and enjoy!
2. If you want, you can add some protein.
3. Enjoy!

Alkaline Ginger Soup

Nutrition and simplicity very often go hand in hand. This soup is great not only as an easy dinner recipe, but also as a side dish or nourishing, alkaline tonic.

Serves: 4
Ingredients:
- 10 carrots, peeled and chopped
- 1 onion, diced
- 4 tablespoons minced ginger
- 3 cups vegetable broth
- 2 tablespoons coconut oil
- Himalayan salt and black pepper to taste

Instructions:
1. Heat up some coconut oil in a large pan (medium heat) and fry until translucent.
2. Reduce the heat to low heat, add carrots and ginger. Keep stirring.
3. Now add vegetable broth, and simmer until carrots are tender.
4. When done, place through a blender.
5. You can serve it with some protein of your choice.
6. It's great in winter, but you can also serve it cold, as a summer refreshment.

Alkaline Mineral Broth

Another amazing mix of common-sense superfoods in a common-sense recipe. There is no need to splurge on exotic superfoods that are very often hard to pronounce and to find. I recently recommended this recipe in one of my newsletters, and the feedback I got was amazing. If you want to receive more recipes from me (as soon as they are created or as soon as I discover them), remember to join our alkaline wellness club (free newsletter) at: www.bitly.com/AlkalineMarta

Serves: 6

Ingredients:
- 4 medium sweet potatoes
- 1 cup zucchini, chopped
- 1 cup cabbage, chopped
- 1 cup celery, chopped
- 5 carrots, chopped
- 1 cup collard greens, chopped
- 1 cup kale, chopped
- ½ cup onion, minced
- 1/2 cup parsley
- ½ cup beets
- 5 cloves garlic
- ½ cup flax seeds
- A few inches of ginger root
- Himalayan salt, olive oil and black pepper to taste
- 3 liters of water
- Optional: Any other veggies you have around the house.

Instructions:
1. Place the veggies in a big pot and add water.
2. Bring to boil using low heat and simmer 4 hours or more.
3. Add Himalayan salt, olive oil and spices.
4. Strain and keep the broth.
5. Drink at least 1 cup per day.
6. Variations: If you like thicker soups instead of broths, you can blend everything together in a blender.
7. In case you decide to strain it, you can keep the veggies for curry stir-fries and vegetable pancakes.

Alkaline Thai Style Potatoes

Great recipe for those who love Asian flavors!

Serves: 3

Ingredients:

- 3 medium sized sweet potatoes or yams
- ½ cup coconut milk
- ¼ cup smooth almond butter (raw, unsweetened)
- 1 tablespoon wheat free tamari sauce
- 1 tablespoon chili sauce
- 1 teaspoon olive oil
- ½ teaspoon red pepper flakes
- 2 minced garlic cloves
- 2-3 drops liquid stevia
- Pinch of Himalayan salt
- 2 tablespoons coconut oil
- 1 cup chickpeas, cooked and drained
- 1 red bell pepper, chopped
- ¼ teaspoon garlic powder
- Salt and pepper, to taste
- 2 green onions, finely chopped

Garnish:

- 1 tbsp. cilantro, finely chopped
- ¼ chopped cashews

Instructions:

1. Preheat oven to 400 degrees Fahrenheit (200 Celsius).
2. Make several holes with a knife or fork in each sweet potato. Bake in the oven for an hour or an hour and fifteen minutes, wrapped tightly in foil.
3. In the meantime, blend together garlic clove, red pepper, olive oil, garlic sauce, tamari sauce, coconut milk and almond butter using a food processor or a blender. Add 2-3 drops of stevia to sweeten.
4. Pour some coconut oil into a sauté pan using medium heat and add red pepper, onions, chickpeas as well as salt and pepper. Sauté for 5 minutes.
5. Turn off the heat when soft.
6. Fill each half of a sweet potato with mixture, garnish with cilantro and cashews. Enjoy!

Alkaline Couscous

This is a very simple solution for busy people and the dinner leftovers can make a great take-away lunch for the next day!

Serves: 2
Ingredients:

- 1 cup couscous (preferably gluten-free)
- 1 yellow onion, peeled
- 1 cucumber
- 4 tomatoes
- 1/2 red chili
- ¼ cup fresh mint leaves
- ¼ cup fresh coriander leaves
- 1/4 cup fresh parsley leaves
- 1 /2 cup pureed tomato
- 2 tablespoons olive oil
- 1 small lemon, juice and zest
- 1 teaspoon ground cumin
- 1 teaspoon paprika
- Himalayan salt to taste
- powdered black pepper
- boiling water

Instructions:

1. Place couscous in a big bowl.
2. Add enough boiling water to cover the couscous. Be careful not to add too much water.
3. Stir in some salt and spices. Cover and set aside.
4. In the meantime, chop the veggies (onion, tomatoes, and chili) and herbs (parsley, coriander and mint).
5. Now take a couscous bowl and stir in the tomato puree until well coated.
6. Add all the veggies, herbs and spices mixing well.
7. Sprinkle over some olive oil, lemon zest and juice, and add salt and pepper.

Easy Root Salad

This is yet another delicious, easy to make, vegan friendly option that is fantastic for detoxification. It can make a simple dish if you are not too hungry, or serve as a side dish.

Serves: 2
Ingredients:
- 4 fresh beetroots, peeled and sliced thinly
- 3 carrots, peeled and spiraled
- 1 heart celery, with leaves, sliced
- ½ cup arugula
- ½ cup radishes, diced
- 1 fennel bulb, (save the roots for later use)
- Olive oil and lemon juice or alkaline chili dressing (see recipe below)
- Himalayan salt and black pepper

Instructions:
1. Place beets, celery heart and leaves, radishes, arugula and fennel in a salad bowl.
2. Toss well and sprinkle over some lemon juice and olive oil (or alkaline chili dressing from the next recipe).
3. Season with Himalayan salt and pepper. Enjoy!

Alkaline Chili Dressing

This simple recipe is a great way to spice up all your salads, dips, sauces and even wraps.

Ingredients:
- 2 red chilies (fresh, not dried)
- 1/2 cup extra virgin olive oil
- 3 tablespoons lemon juice
- 1 tablespoon lime juice
- 1/4 cup fresh mint leaves, leaves picked and finely chopped
- A few tablespoons coconut milk
- Himalayan salt
- Black pepper

Instructions:
1. Peel the chilies; take out and discard the seeds.
2. Finely chop the chilies and combine with lemon juice, coconut milk, mint and olive oil.
3. Add salt and pepper to taste.
4. Sprinkle a bit to your regular salad dressing. Careful, it's hot!

Easy Sweet Potato Curry

This recipe is a real pleasure for your taste buds!

Serves: 2

Ingredients:

- 1 cup chickpeas, cooked and drained
- 2 tbsp. olive or coconut oil
- 4 medium sized sweet potatoes, peeled and cubed
- 1 onion, diced
- 1 tbsp. ginger powder
- 1 tbsp. curry powder
- ½ cup vegetable stock
- 1 can full fat coconut milk
- salt and pepper to taste

To garnish:

A handful of cilantro and mint leaves

To serve:

Arugula, spinach or other greens to serve on side.

Instructions:

1. Add 1 tbsp. olive or coconut oil to a skillet and heat up on medium-high heat.
2. Add the onions and cook until translucent.
3. Reduce to low/medium heat and add ginger, garlic and curry powder, and pinch of Himalayan salt cooking for another 2 minutes.
4. Now add the potatoes and vegetable stock. Keep stirring.
5. When almost soft, add chickpeas and coconut milk. Stir again. Turn off the heat when potatoes are done.
6. Garnish with cilantro and mint leaves and serve with some greens on side.
7. Enjoy!

Alkaline Tacos

This vegan friendly recipe combines the amazing benefits of black beans (high in fiber and vegan protein) and broccoli (great for liver detoxification, just like all green foods). While very few people are naturally attracted to broccoli, this recipe makes it more appealing.

Serves: 2-4
Ingredients:
Broccoli:

- 1 large head of broccoli, sliced into small florets
- 3 tbsp. olive oil
- salt and pepper to taste

Black Beans:

- 1 tbsp. olive oil
- 1 white onion, finely chopped
- 2 garlic cloves, minced
- 2 tbsp. organic tomato sauce
- ¾ cup black beans, cooked and rinsed
- 2 cups vegetable broth (you can use alkaline mineral broth from previous recipes)
- 1 tsp. ground cumin
- ½ tsp. chili powder

Tacos:

- 8 gluten-free tortillas

Taco Sauce:

- 1/3 cup vegan mayonnaise (check out the bonus recipes at the end of this book)
- 2 tbsp. lemon juice
- 3 tbsp. hot sauce of your choice
- salt and pepper to taste

Instructions:

1. Preheat oven to 400 degrees Fahrenheit (about 200 Celsius).
2. Massage broccoli with some coconut oil.
3. Add salt and pepper to taste, and place broccoli on a big baking dish.
4. Roast until golden brown (about 30 minutes). Remove once half way through to turn.
5. In the meantime, take a sauté pan, heat some coconut oil over medium heat and add onion and garlic.
6. Season with a pinch of salt, and cook for a few minutes until soft.
7. Add tomato paste, cumin and chili powder. Stir well.
8. Now add black beans and veggie broth.
9. Simmer for 10 minutes so that the beans take the flavor.
10. In the meantime, whisk all the sauce ingredients together and set aside.
11. Once everything is done, prepare for serving. Top each tortilla with black bean mixture and broccoli. Sprinkle over some sauce and enjoy!

Easy Cucumber Bean Salad

Great salad recipe for hot summers, or as a side dish throughout the year.

Serves: 2
Ingredients:

- 2 medium large cucumbers, peeled and sliced (or spiraled)
- 2 carrots
- 2 big ripe tomatoes
- 1 red or green bell pepper, finely chopped
- 1 cup red onions, diced
- ½ cup cilantro, finely chopped
- ½ cup cashews
- ½ cup garbanzo beans, cooked and drained
- ½ tsp. Himalayan salt
- ½ tsp. garlic powder
- ½ tsp. chili powder
- ¼ tsp. ginger powder
- ¼ tsp. cumin
- 1/8 tsp. turmeric
- Cilantro leaves to garnish
- Juice of 1 small lime

Instructions:

1. Mix all the salad ingredients in a big salad bowl.
2. Toss well adding spices, salt and olive oil.
3. Sprinkle over some lime juice. Garnish with fresh cilantro leaves.
4. Serve and enjoy!

White Bean Avocado Sandwich

This recipe is a great "vegan fast-food" option with an alkaline twist. It also works well for lunch. It's not that you have to quit bread forever. Just choose healthy bread options (for example gluten-free, multi-grain) and of course, don't overdo it.

Serves: 2
Ingredients:
- ½ cup white beans, mashed
- 2 tbsp. olive oil
- Pinch of Himalayan salt and black pepper
- 4 slices of multi-grain or gluten free bread (wraps also work great)
- A few onion rings
- 1 carrot, peeled and thinly sliced
- 1 avocado, peeled, pitted and thinly sliced
- 2 handfuls of sprouts (alfalfa or soy sprouts - you decide)

Instructions:
1. Lay your bread slices or wraps of choice open, and add some bean mixture.
2. Top with onion rings, carrots, sprouts and avocado.
3. Close your sandwiches, serve and enjoy!

Easy Quinoa Bowl

This recipe combines the alkalizing benefits of avocado (excellent source of healthy fats) and kale (which is high in Vitamins K, A and C.)

Serves: 4

- 1 cup quinoa, cooked
- 1 bunch kale stems removed and finely chopped
- ½ cup lemon juice
- 2 tbsp. olive oil
- ½ jalapeno pepper, diced
- ½ tsp. cumin
- salt to taste

Avocado salsa:

- 1 avocado, sliced
- 2 tomato, chopped
- 1 jalapeno pepper, diced
- ½ cup cilantro leaves, chopped
- ¼-1/2 red onion, finely chopped
- 1 lemon, juiced

Instructions:

1. Prepare your dressing by whisking together lemon juice, olive oil, jalapeno, cumin and salt.
2. Place kale leaves in a salad bowl and massage it well with your salad dressing.
3. In a separate bowl, mix together all avocado salsa ingredients and set aside.
4. In serving bowls, distribute equal amounts of quinoa and kale.
5. Top with avocado salsa.
6. Enjoy!

Alkaline Spinach Soup
Great for a well-deserved liver detox!

Serves: 4-5
Ingredients:
- 2 tbsp. coconut oil
- 2 leeks, white parts, chopped
- 4 garlic cloves, peeled and minced
- 4 celery stalks, chopped
- 3 medium heads of broccoli, chopped
- 8 cups of veggie broth
- 3 cups spinach leaves, chopped
- 1 cup parsley, chopped
- salt and pepper to taste

Instructions:
1. Heat some coconut oil in a pot over medium heat.
2. Add garlic and leeks, and fry until just slightly browned.
3. Add broccoli and celery, stirring for a few minutes.
4. Now add vegetable stock and bring everything to a boil on low heat.
5. Remove from heat when broccoli gets tender.
6. Then, add the spinach and parsley, just to heat it slightly.
7. Place the mixture through a food processor and blend until smooth.
8. Season to taste, serve and enjoy. Personally, I love it creamy, with some coconut oil.

Amazing Raw Tomato Soup

This recipe is super easy and you can also enjoy it between your meals for more alkaline energy!

Serves: 4-6
Ingredients

- 6 big tomatoes, peeled
- 2 carrots
- 1 inch fresh ginger, peeled
- 3 garlic cloves, minced
- 2 tablespoons olive oil
- 1/2 cup vegetable broth
- ½ cup coconut milk (full fat)
- Salt and fresh pepper to taste

Instructions:

1. Blend all the ingredients in a food processor or a blender.
2. Serve raw or slightly warmed.
3. Personally, I like to throw in some stir-fried veggies, chickpeas or quinoa.
4. This recipe is highly alkalizing and so if you decide to eat something that is not alkaline (for example meat), it's always good to have it as a side dish to achieve alkaline balance.

Raw Spinach Salad

Spinach is miraculous and if you are serious about going alkaline, you should consider eating more of it. This recipe helps you do it in an easy and enjoyable way.

Serves: 4-6
Ingredients:
- ¼ cup strawberries, halved
- 8 cups spinach leaves, washed and chopped thinly
- 4 tbsp. almonds, crushed
- ½ onion, finely chopped
- 1 grapefruit, peeled and chopped (sprinkle over some stevia if you find it hard to eat grapefruit)
- 1 avocado, peeled, pitted and chopped
- 2 tablespoons chia seeds for more nutrition
- Olive oil and Himalayan salt to taste

Instructions:
1. In a salad bowl, combine all the salad ingredients and stir well.
2. Sprinkle over some olive oil and Himalayan salt.
3. Enjoy!

Alkaline Thai Kale Salad

This simple recipe is an easy and delicious way to sneak more kale into your diet.

Serves: 4
Ingredients:

- 3 cups kale leaves, stemmed
- 1 large sized red onion, thinly sliced
- 2 tablespoons coconut aminos
- Juice of 2 limes
- ½ cup coconut milk
- 2 jalapeño peepers, diced
- Zest of 1 lime
- 2 orange sweet peppers, diced
- 3 cloves garlic, peeled, minced
- Coconut oil

Instructions:

1. Sauté the red onion slices in some coconut oil.
2. Add the garlic clove, sweet peppers and jalapeño slices to the onions.
3. Stir fry until slightly golden.
4. Blanch the kale leaves in a pot of boiling water. Drain and set aside.
5. In the meantime, mix the coconut aminos, lime zest and lime juice with the coconut milk. Set aside.
6. Mix kale leaves and the veggies. Drizzle the coconut milk dressing on top to serve.
7. Enjoy!

Apple and Celery Root Salad

Apples in salads are great and make it much tastier!

Serves: 2-4
Ingredients:
- 1 medium red apple, peeled and diced
- 2 tablespoons of *vegan or* home-made mayonnaise (recipe in the bonus section)
- 1 medium sized celery root, peeled and grated
- 4 tablespoons of chopped almonds
- Juice of 1 lemon
- 2 carrots, sliced
- 2 cucumbers, sliced
- 2 tablespoons of coconut cream
- 1/4th cup of minced fresh parsley leaves
- Olive oil and lime juice
- Himalayan salt and pepper to taste

Instructions:
1. Combine all the salad ingredients in a salad bowl.
2. Toss well. Stir in some mayonnaise and give it a thorough mix again.
3. Sprinkle over some olive oil and lime juice.
4. Season with Himalayan salt and black pepper to taste.
5. Enjoy!

Artichoke Salad

Artichokes are miraculous and really good for your liver. They also make delicious salads!

Serves: 2

Ingredients:

- 2-3 brine dipped artichoke hearts, halved
- 2 cups of fresh arugula leaves
- ½ cup of almond powder mixed with cashew powder
- 1 red onion, sliced
- Half cup soy sprouts

Dressing:

- A few tablespoons homemade mayonnaise check the recipe in the bonus section)
- 2 tablespoons olive oil
- Juice of half a lemon

Instructions:

1. Combine all the salad ingredients in a salad bowl.
2. Toss well. Stir in some mayonnaise and give it a thorough mix again.
3. Sprinkle over some olive oil and lime juice.
4. Season with Himalayan salt and black pepper to taste.
5. Enjoy!

Summer Veggies Salad

Servings: 2
Ingredients:
- 1 red organic beetroot, peeled and sliced
- 6 radishes, sliced
- 1 orange
- 1/2 of a red onion, peeled and sliced
- Zucchini, sliced or spiraled stir-fried in coconut oil
- optional: 1 small sized kohlrabi, sliced
- 1 red pepper, deseeded and sliced
- ¼ cup of almonds

Dressing:
- 2-3 tablespoons olive oil
- 2 teaspoons of fresh oregano, chopped
- 1 clove of garlic, peeled and finely chopped
- 2 drops liquid stevia
- 2 tablespoons coconut milk
- 1 tablespoon of fresh parsley leaves, chopped
- Fresh juice of 1 lemon
- Pinch of Himalayan salt

Instructions:
1. Combine all the dressing ingredients, stir well and set aside.
2. Combine all the salad ingredients in a salad bowl.
3. Toss well and sprinkle generously with the salad dressing.
4. Enjoy!

Green Papaya Salad

Papaya is great for digestion and has a plethora of anti-inflammatory benefits. I remember visiting the Canary Islands and indulging in papaya smoothies and salads there because papaya was really cheap and easy to get. I wish I was there now. Holidays are always too short, right?

Serves: 2
Ingredients:
- Cup of mixed fresh lettuce leaves of your choice
- Green papaya, julienned
- ¼ cup radish slices
- A few tablespoons of raw cashew nuts
- ½ cup cherry tomatoes

Spicy Dressing:
- 1 tablespoon maple syrup
- 2 tablespoons of coconut milk or almond milk
- 1 red long chili, seeded and finely chopped
- Juice of 2 limes
- 1 small clove of garlic, peeled and minced

Instructions:
1. Mix all the dressing ingredients in a small bowl and set aside.
2. In the meantime, combine all the salad ingredients in a larger salad bowl.
3. Toss well. Stir in some spicy dressing depending on your taste preferences and give it a thorough mix again.
4. Sprinkle over some olive oil and lime juice.
5. Season with Himalayan salt and black pepper to taste.
6. Enjoy!

Grapefruit Avocado Salad

Both grapefruits and avocados are considered super alkaline foods. Imagine the combined energy powers...

Serves: 4
Ingredients:
- 2 whole avocados, peeled, pitted and sliced
- 2 tablespoons of extra virgin olive oil
- A pinch of Himalayan salt
- ¼ cup almond powder or crashed almonds
- 2 grapefruits, peeled and sliced
- A few raisins (optional)

Instructions:
1. Combine all the salad ingredients in a salad bowl.
2. Toss well. Sprinkle over some olive oil.
3. Season with Himalayan salt.
4. Enjoy! This salad is extremely alkaline and will help you balance your ph level.

Easy Pomegranate Salad

Pomegranates are highly alkalizing fruits and taste great in salads.

Serves: 2
Ingredients:
- 1/2 cup of fresh rocket leaves
- Juice of 1/2 fresh lemon
- 2 oranges, peeled and halved horizontally
- A few tablespoons cashew powder
- 1 whole pomegranate, seeded
- A few small sprigs of mint, leaves separated
- Some olive oil

Instructions:
1. Combine all the salad ingredients in a salad bowl.
2. Toss well.
3. Sprinkle over some olive oil and lemon juice.
4. Enjoy!

SECTION II
Paleo and Vegetarian Alkaline-Friendly Recipes

Simple Chia Seeds Coconut Salmon

Salmon is a great source of vitamin B12, vitamin D, and selenium as well as niacin, omega-3 fatty acids, protein, phosphorus, and vitamin B6. When combined with lots of green veggies, it creates an easy, alkaline-paleo friendly, balanced meal that is also fantastic for weight loss efforts. My grandma was right - if you want to lose weight, eat more fish with veggies!

Chia seeds add to nutritional side of this dish, actually chia seeds are one of the most nutritious foods ever.

Serves: 2-3
Ingredients:

- 2 salmon fillets (6 oz. each)
- 1 tbsp. coconut flour
- 2 tbsps. fresh or dried parsley
- 1 tbsp. olive oil
- 1 tbsp. gluten free mustard
- Himalayan Salt and pepper to taste
- 2-3 tbsps. chia seeds
- 2 cups spinach, washed and chopped
- 1 tablespoon coconut oil
- Half an onion, cut in rings
- ¼ cup coconut milk (thick) for the spinach + a few tablespoons for the salmon

Instructions:

1. Preheat oven to 450 degrees Fahrenheit (230 Celsius).
2. Place salmon on parchment lined baking sheet.
3. Sprinkle over some olive oil.
4. While the oven is getting ready, take a small bowl and mix together coconut flour, parsley, salt and pepper.
5. Sprinkle onto the salmon and pour over a few

tablespoons of coconut milk.

6. Bake for about 10-15 minutes.
7. While the salmon is getting ready, prepare the spinach. Start by heating up some coconut oil in a frying pan.
8. Add onion rings and fry on medium heat until translucent.
9. Reduce the heat to low heat and add the spinach. Stir well and pour over ¼ cup of coconut milk.
10. Add a bit of Himalayan salt and pepper. Cook until spinach is soft.
11. Serve with baked salmon and sprinkle over some chia seeds.
12. Enjoy!

Easy Yummy Spinach Salad

Quick and easy detox recipe with amazing anti-inflammatory nutrients from fruit, veggies, and protein.

Serves: 2

Ingredients:

- 2 cups spinach leaves, chopped
- 1 avocado, peeled, pitted and sliced
- 1 peach, pitted and chopped
- 1 cup tomatoes, sliced
- ½ cup almonds
- 2-4 slices smoked salmon, chopped
- 2 tablespoon olive oil
- Juice of ½ lemon
- Himalayan salt and black pepper

Instructions:

1. Mix everything well in a large bowl.
2. Sprinkle over some olive oil and lemon juice.
3. Season with Himalayan salt and black pepper.

Easy Vegetarian Pizza (Vegetarian, Paleo)

This recipe is a delicious pizza alternative made with almond flour. It's gluten-free, and paleo friendly. Even though eggs are not the most alkaline ingredients, this recipe is nicely balanced thanks to a variety of alkalizing veggies on top. It's a great treat that will not spoil your alkaline efforts. Eat it totally guilt-free.

Serves: 4
Ingredients:
Pizza Crust:

- 4 organic eggs
- 4 cups almond flour
- 4 tbsp. olive oil
- 1 tsp. Himalayan salt

Topping:

- ½ cup tomato paste
- 1 bunch basil leaves and/or oregano
- 2 tomatoes, chopped
- 3-4 cloves garlic, minced
- 1 onion, chopped
- 1 red pepper, sliced
- 1 green pepper, sliced
- Optional (not alkaline and not paleo but OK as an occasional treat)- parmesan or mozzarella cheese; you could also substitute for vegan cheese

Instructions:

1. Preheat oven to 350 degrees Fahrenheit (or 175 Celsius).
2. To prepare crust, simply mix all the crust ingredients until you have a thick, sticky dough.
3. Spread olive oil over a large piece of parchment paper.
4. Roll your dough out until desired thickness, personally, I like it medium, not too thick, not too thin.
5. If you have a pizza tray, move parchment paper and pizza to it. You can also use flat baking.

6. Bake for about 10 minutes, until the middle of the crust is cooked through.
7. Remove from the oven for a few minutes and add your toppings (veggies and spices). As a treat, you can also add some cheese (not alkaline though).
8. Put back in the oven for another 10 minutes, (maximum 15 minutes) until veggies get soft.
9. Serve with some greens on side. Enjoy!

Cucumber Tuna Salad (Alkaline-Paleo)

A very simple way to conjure up a quick dinner salad! Tune is not alkaline, but the recipe is nicely balanced by green, alkaline ingredients. If you feel like grain-free, this is a meal for you.

Serves: 4

Ingredients:

- 2 cans organic tuna
- 3 cucumbers, peeled and sliced
- 1/2 red onion, thinly sliced
- 3 tbsp. lime juice
- 2 tablespoons olive oil
- 3 tbsp. coconut yoghurt or coconut cream (thick coconut milk is also fine)
- Himalayan salt and pepper to taste
- 2 avocados, peeled, pitted and sliced
- ½ cup blueberries
- 1 tsp. chopped cilantro

Instructions:

1. Whisk or thoroughly stir together all ingredients in a bowl.
2. Sprinkle over some lime juice, coconut yoghurt and olive oil.
3. Mix well, season with salt and pepper and enjoy!

Baked Swordfish with Mango Salsa

Fantastic, alkaline-paleo friendly recipe for those who wish to add more variety to their diets.

Servings: 4

Ingredients:
- 4 (6-ounce) boneless swordfish steaks
- Olive oil, or coconut oil
- ½ cup chopped pineapple
- ½ small red pepper, cored and chopped
- ¼ cup diced red onion
- 2 tablespoons freshly squeezed lime juice
- 2 tablespoons chopped cilantro
- 1 ripe mango, pitted and diced
- Himalayan Salt and pepper to taste

Instructions:
1. Preheat the oven to 350°F.(175 °C)
2. Sprinkle the swordfish with olive oil and season with salt and pepper.
3. Place the fillets on a parchment-lined baking sheet.
4. Bake for about 20 minutes.
5. In the meantime, take a medium bowl and combine the mango, pineapple, red pepper and onion adding in the lime juice, cilantro, salt and pepper.
6. Serve the swordfish steaks hot topped with the mango salsa from the step 5. I suggest you serve it with some big green salad on side to create a really balanced, nutritious and alkaline-friendly meal.
7. Enjoy!

Alkaline Pesto Pasta with Veggies

Zucchini noodles are just fantastic and a great option on gluten-free, grain-free diets. This recipe is light and refreshing, perfect for hot summer evenings. Really alkalizing. You can never go wrong with this one.

Serves: 4
Ingredients:
Pesto:

- 2 cups fresh basil
- ¼ cup freshly grated parmesan cheese (optional, you can very well do without it or you can use vegan cheese instead).
- ½ cup olive oil
- juice of half a lemon
- 1/3 cup pine or walnuts
- 3 garlic cloves
- salt and pepper to taste

Veggie Pasta

- 2 cups zucchini, spiraled into noodles
- Coconut oil

Instructions:

1. First, prepare pesto sauce. Begin by toasting pine or walnuts, heat a bit of olive oil in a pan on medium heat, add nuts, and stir constantly until browned. Remove from heat.
2. Add all pesto ingredients to a food processor and blend until smooth.
3. Season to taste as needed. Set aside.
4. Heat up some coconut oil in a medium-size skillet and add spiraled zucchini. Stir-fry on low/medium heat for about 5 minutes until soft.
5. Pour over the pesto sauce and stir well.
6. Serve and enjoy!

Vegetarian Quinoa Burgers

Quinoa doesn't have to be boring. You can use this amazing gluten-free super grain to conjure up amazing burgers that your whole family will adore!

Serves: 4
Ingredients:
- 1 cup black beans, cooked and rinsed
- ¼ cup quinoa, cooked
- ½ cup alkaline water
- ½ cup ground flax seeds
- ½ cup bell pepper, finely chopped
- ¼ cup onion, finely chopped
- 2 garlic cloves, minced
- 1 tsp. chili sauce
- 1 organic egg
- 3 tbsp. coconut oil
- 2 tsp. ground cumin
- ½ tsp. Himalayan salt

Instructions:
1. Place black beans through a food processor until smooth.
2. Put in a mash bowl and add cooked quinoa, garlic, bell pepper, onion, flax meal, cumin, hot sauce, and egg.
3. Mix well.
4. Start forming patties (expect 4-5). Set aside.
5. Heat some coconut oil in a pan (use medium heat).
6. Cook the patties on both sides (about 2-3 minutes per each side) about 3 minutes per side.
7. Serve your crispy burgers with heaps of green salads. Leftovers will also make a great takeaway lunch for next day.
8. Enjoy!

Bonus Recipes

Homemade Mayo
Vegetarian Option:

Mix: 1 organic egg yolk with a pinch of Himalaya salt, half teaspoon of Dijon mustard, 1 tablespoon of lemon juice and a few drops of white vinegar and half cup of avocado oil or coconut oil. Enjoy!

Vegan Option:

Mix: half cup almond or coconut milk, 2 tablespoons fresh lemon juice, 1 tablespoon Dijon mustard, half cup of olive oil, pinch of salt and pepper. You can experiment with the consistency by adding some almond powder and coconut oil. Enjoy!

Alkaline Yummy Coconut Macaroons

These are dangerously addictive and really healthy. Perfect for evening time when you have an after-dinner "sweet tooth." Coconut is an alkaline fruit and spices like cinnamon and vanilla not only add to your wellbeing but also have anti-inflammatory and soothing properties. You don't need to feel guilty about this one.

Ingredients:

- 1 cup coconut butter (may be hard to find, but not impossible, I get my from health store or from Amazon.com)
- 1 cups shredded, unsweetened coconut
- A few drops if liquid stevia
- 1 tsp. vanilla
- dash of cinnamon and nutmeg

Instructions:

1. Preheat oven to 325 degrees Fahrenheit (160 Celsius), and line a baking sheet with parchment paper.
2. Heat the coconut butter (low heat and small pot) stirring energetically so that it's completely melted.
3. Mix all ingredients together in a bowl, until well combined.
4. Dough should be thick, you can always add a bit more shredded coconut to make it thicker.
5. Form small cookies and place them on the baking sheet.
6. Bake for about 15 minutes (keep checking as these are easy to burn so don't leave them unattended).
7. Allow your macaroons to cool for 20 minutes, serve and enjoy.

Chia Flax Dessert

This is a great, guilt-free dessert option for you to enjoy. Everyone loves chocolate and this recipe is a healthy, dairy-free and gluten-free alternative that is totally compatible with the alkaline diet.

Serves: 1-2
Ingredients:
- 1 cup berries (organic if possible)
- 1 ½ cup coconut milk
- 1 tbsp. chia seeds, ground
- 1 tbsp. flax seeds, ground
- 1 tsp. unsweetened cocoa powder
- 2 drops liquid stevia
- 1 tsp. cinnamon

Instructions:
1. Blend using a blender and enjoy!
2. Serve immediately or chill in a fridge.

Conclusion

Thank you for reading!

I hope that with so many alkaline-friendly recipes you will be motivated and inspired to start your journey towards vibrant health and total wellbeing.

Remember, the beauty of incorporating alkaline foods into your daily diet is that you are making simple, yet sustainable changes that will work for your wellness long-term.

In reducing processed foods from your diet, you are working to prevent many potential diseases such as cancer, diabetes, arthritis and many more. On top of that, you are providing your family with important nutritional foundation that they need to create a life full of happiness, energy and fulfilment.

If you enjoyed my book, it would be greatly appreciated if you left a review so others can receive the same benefits you have. Your review can help other people take this important step to take care of their health and inspire them to start a new chapter in their lives.

At the same time, you can help me serve you and all my other readers even more.

I'd be thrilled to hear from you. I would love to know your top 3 recipes.

Simply visit the link below or go to your Amazon orders and write a short review to share your experience. I know you are busy and I would like to thank you in advance for considering taking a couple of minutes to review this book.

Link (amazon US): www.amazon.com/author/mtuchowska

Honestly, whenever I get a review, I jump around like a little kid and I read it all over again, my cheeks rosy with excitement!

Even when I get a meaningful, negative review with constructive criticism I feel grateful and I take immediate action to improve my work to serve my readers the best I can.

It's all about constant progress, both in health, life and professional career.

Have a fantastic day,
I wish you all the best on your journey

Marta Tuchowska

www.HolisticWellnessProject.com
www.AlkalineDietLifestyle.com

ADDITIONAL RESOURCES FOR ALKALINE WELLNESS MOTIVATION

Looking for more recipes and wellness?

Follow me on Instagram and discover my holistic lifestyle secrets + dozens of alkaline recipes, picks and motivational videos that will help you keep on track throughout the day:

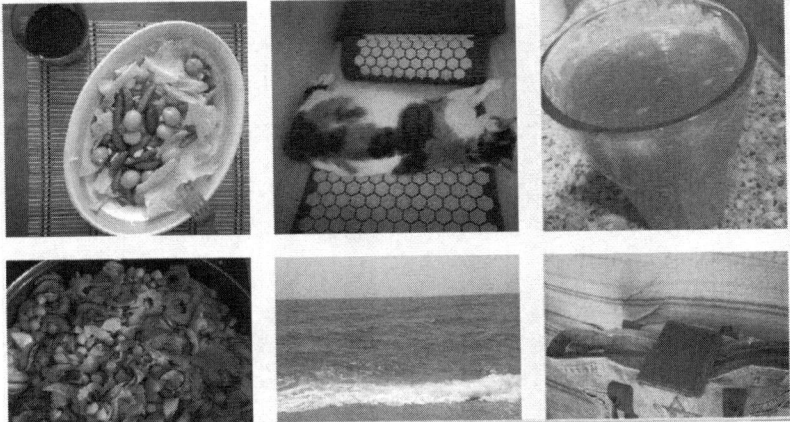

www.instagram.com/Marta_Wellness

Free eBook

Don't forget to download your free copy of
"Revolutionize Your Life with Alkaline Foods"
Download Link:
www.holisticwellnessproject.com/alkaline-diet-ebook/giveaway.html

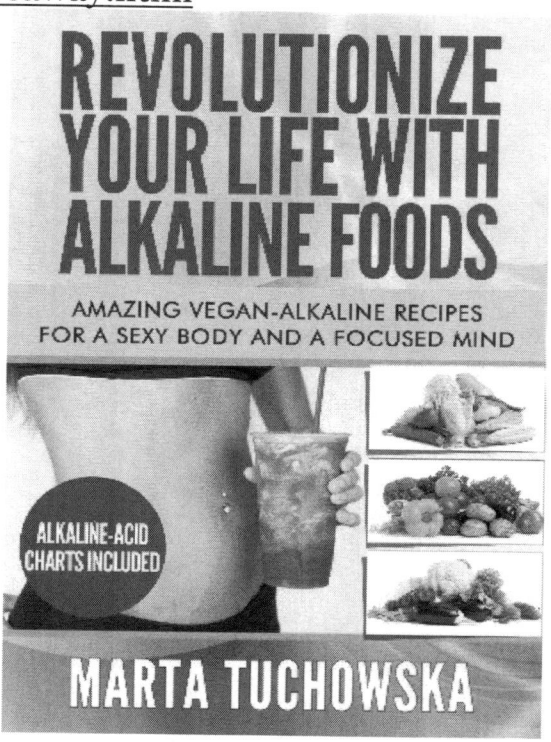

Let Me Help You

If you have any questions, doubts, or you find my instructions confusing and need more guidance, please e-mail me and ask for a free consultation. I am here to help. Don't be shy. I am also looking for feedback. If you have any suggestions that can help me improve my work, please let me know and I will take an immediate action to serve you better in the next editions. Thanks and have a fantastic day!

info@holisticwellnessproject.com

More Wellness Books from Marta Tuchowska (available in all Amazon stores, simply search for "Marta Tuchowska")

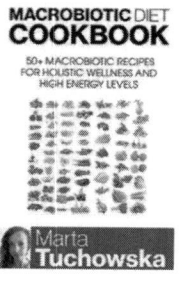 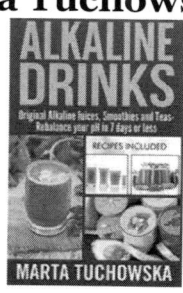 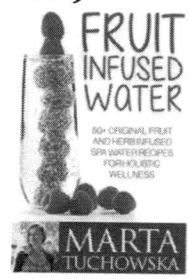

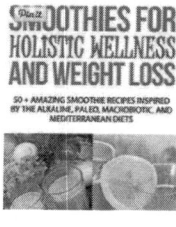 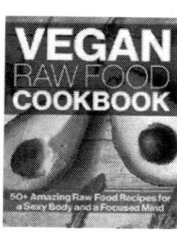 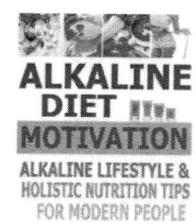

1. Amazon.com link:
   www.amazon.com/author/mtuchowska

2. Blog link:
   www.holisticwellnessproject.com/personal-development-books/alkaline-diet

FINALLY- LET'S KEEP IN TOUCH:

www.instagram.com/Marta_Wellness
www.facebook.com/HolisticWellnessProject
www.twitter.com/Marta_Wellness
www.pinterest.com/martaWellness/
www.udemy.com/u/martatuchowska
www.linkedin.com/in/martatuchowska
www.plus.google.com/+MartaTuchowska

NEED MORE MOTIVATION?

Listen to my podcast:

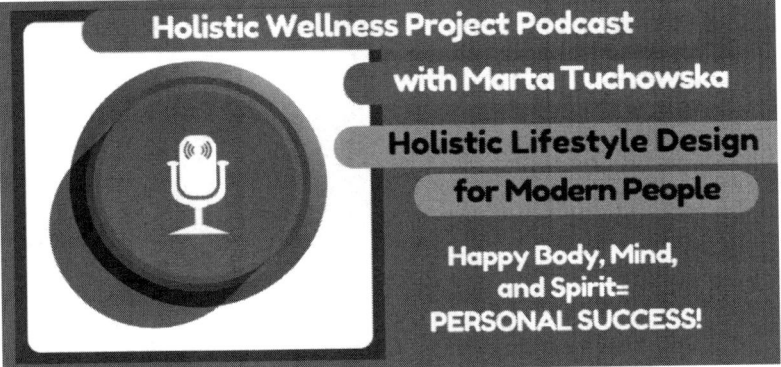

www.holisticwellnessproject.com/blog/podcast
www.holisticwellnessproject.com/blog/alkaline-diet
->most of my articles are **also available in MP3** so that you can feed your mind with positive information even if you are busy.

I wish you wellness, health, and success in whatever it is that you want to accomplish.
With lots of LOVE and positive energy,

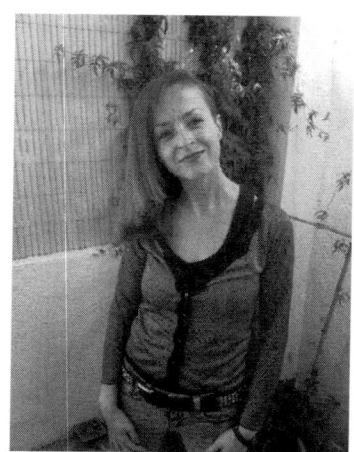

Marta Tuchowska

Made in the USA
Middletown, DE
19 January 2016